Laurenţiu Pirtea
Andreea Adriana Jitariu
Marius Raica

AF141887

Angiogenesis and lymphangiogenesis in ovarian cancer

Lessons from the lab to the clinic

LAP LAMBERT Academic Publishing

Impressum / Imprint

Bibliografische Information der Deutschen Nationalbibliothek: Die Deutsche Nationalbibliothek verzeichnet diese Publikation in der Deutschen Nationalbibliografie; detaillierte bibliografische Daten sind im Internet über http://dnb.d-nb.de abrufbar.

Alle in diesem Buch genannten Marken und Produktnamen unterliegen warenzeichen-, marken- oder patentrechtlichem Schutz bzw. sind Warenzeichen oder eingetragene Warenzeichen der jeweiligen Inhaber. Die Wiedergabe von Marken, Produktnamen, Gebrauchsnamen, Handelsnamen, Warenbezeichnungen u.s.w. in diesem Werk berechtigt auch ohne besondere Kennzeichnung nicht zu der Annahme, dass solche Namen im Sinne der Warenzeichen- und Markenschutzgesetzgebung als frei zu betrachten wären und daher von jedermann benutzt werden dürften.

Bibliographic information published by the Deutsche Nationalbibliothek: The Deutsche Nationalbibliothek lists this publication in the Deutsche Nationalbibliografie; detailed bibliographic data are available in the Internet at http://dnb.d-nb.de.

Any brand names and product names mentioned in this book are subject to trademark, brand or patent protection and are trademarks or registered trademarks of their respective holders. The use of brand names, product names, common names, trade names, product descriptions etc. even without a particular marking in this work is in no way to be construed to mean that such names may be regarded as unrestricted in respect of trademark and brand protection legislation and could thus be used by anyone.

Coverbild / Cover image: www.ingimage.com

Verlag / Publisher:
LAP LAMBERT Academic Publishing
ist ein Imprint der / is a trademark of
OmniScriptum GmbH & Co. KG
Heinrich-Böcking-Str. 6-8, 66121 Saarbrücken, Deutschland / Germany
Email: info@lap-publishing.com

Herstellung: siehe letzte Seite /
Printed at: see last page
ISBN: 978-3-659-80103-7

Zugl. / Approved by: Timisoara, University of Medicine and Pharmacy "Victor Babes", Post-doctoral dissertation, 2009

TABLE OF CONTENTS

Author:

Laurențiu Pirtea

Co-authors:

Andreea Adriana Jitariu
Anca Maria Cîmpean
Marius Raica

1. INTRODUCTION

Cancer is currently the most common human condition and has exceeded cardiovascular disease in terms of specific incidence and mortality in the last two years. Unquestionably, remarkable progress in the diagnosis, prognosis and therapy of cancer was made in the last decades, but apparently carcinogenic factors (regardless of their nature) associated with changes in lifestyle, continue to act effectively. Intrinsic causes and natural evolution of the human malignant process are still the subject of numerous controversies, and in this context, effective therapeutic methods are still isolated, with limited effectiveness, associated with more or less significant extension of post-treatment survival expectancy. In the last few years, gene analysis of malignant tumors generated new classifications, with prognostic and especially therapeutic impact. Perhaps the best example is the one regarding hormone-dependent breast cancer, as well as ovarian cancer. This approach has lead to new perspectives not only for research, but also for diagnosis and therapy, initiating for the first time an individually customized treatment approach rather than one addressed to a group of patients.

After the introduction on a wide scale of investigations regarding growth factors and specific receptors, the molecular mechanisms of tumor cell proliferation, local progression and distant metastasis began to be deciphered. New diagnostic, prognostic and therapeutic methods were introduced, and probably the most important acquisition in recent years consists in the targeted therapy based on humanized monoclonal antibodies. But the results of the clinical trials did not confirm each time the observations obtained in vitro and on experimental models. It is not a huge surprise given the insufficient knowledge on the fundamental level on the one hand and the economic interests of the big producers on the other.

Ovarian cancer has been known for a very long time as unpredictable in terms of the natural evolution. There are virtually unknown 'standard' progression and metastasis models as well as a differential and often inconsistent response to the adjuvant anti-cancer therapy. These uncertainties may be explained by insufficient knowledge of the expression of cell growth factor, of the tumor microenvironment and perhaps not least, of angiogenesis and lymphangiogenesis, which have been much less studied in the normal ovary and ovarian tumors than for other tumor locations.

Angiogenesis is the process of new blood vessels formation from existing ones and has proved to be an essential process in development, reproduction and cell proliferation, both in normal and pathological conditions. Tumor angiogenesis has some specific features and sequential mechanisms, also known as the angiogenic switch, that have already been exploited by means of therapy. Antiangiogenic medication is accepted nowadays as adjunctive anti-cancer therapy in a wide variety of human tumors. Much less data is known about ovarian tumors specific angiogenesis compared to malignant lesions developed in other anatomical regions. Initially it was assumed that from this point of view, ovarian carcinoma behaves like other tumors in this category - but this hypothesis proved to be false. Accordingly, the results of clinical trials based on antiangiogenic medication in ovarian cancer have been disappointing. In addition, unlike other sites of cancer, in ovarian cancer not all links in the proangiogenic chain have yet been explored and the expression of many of the growth factors involved in this process, as well as specific receptor expression are virtually unknown. For these reasons, there are currently no predictive markers for the response to antiangiogenic or antivascular therapy in ovarian cancers. One aspect that is not to be neglected, but that was very little studied in ovarian tumors is the tumor-associated lymphangiogenesis and its clinical significance. Data on these issues are even fewer, and their clinical significance is unknown.

In the present study we aimed to study tumor angiogenesis and lymphangiogenesis aspects, in the hope that we will succeed to specify their prognostic value and characterize a number of new potential therapeutic targets. This work could not have been accomplished without the collaboration between the Histology and Gynecology Departments of "Victor Babeş" University Timişoara, and in this way I bring thanks to the colleagues from both departments for contributing with cases, for morphological and immunohistochemical staining processing which allowed the following interpretations and conclusions. I would also like to express my gratitude towards the management of "Victor Babeş" University Timişoara for providing the propitious environment, essential in carrying out this work.

2. ANGIOGENESIS AND LYMPHANGIOGENESIS IN OVARIAN CANCER-FACTS AND CONTROVERSIES

Angiogenesis represents the development of new blood vessels from existing ones. This process is an essential component for the growth and development of any solid tumor or metastases. Tumor cells express certain angiogenic factors suggesting that tumors develop their own blood supply from the host endothelium. Angiogenesis is the stimulation of new endothelial cell formation and the development of new blood vessels (Sharma et al., 2001). Without the support of neoformation vessels, tumor expansion would not exceed 1-2 mm, because tumor growth is strictly dependent on the nutritional support offered by them. In the absence of angiogenesis, the evolution of the tumoral formation would be towards necrosis and apoptosis. Thus it can be advocated that angiogenesis has a crucial role in tumor progression. The triggering of the angiogenesis process marks the start of the rapid tumor proliferative phase, local and subsequently distant invasion. Angiogenesis plays an important role in malignant transformation of premalignant and borderline lesions. Immature neoformation vessels with an increased permeability of the basal membrane facilitate the passage of tumor cells in the blood and lymphatic stream, hence facilitating the metastasis process (Folkman et al., 1989). Normal cells that transform into tumor cells are not potentially angiogenic. Experimental studies on spontaneous tumors in transgenic mice have shown that the acquisition of the angiogenic phenotype is a discrete event which takes place during the progressive stages of tumorgenesis, starting with the pre-malignant stage. Many human tumors are detected by mammography, but at that point the tumor is already vascularized. On the other hand, many tumors arise without angiogenic activity, remain in the state of ISC (in situ carcinoma) for a long period of time and then gain angiogenic phenotype. Thus, the angiogenic phenotype appears after the expression of the malignant phenotype in the majority of primary tumors. There are exceptions, as seen in malignant cervical lesions, in which the stage of dysplasia becomes neovascularized prior to tumor development. The sequence of these events has been also demonstrated in some spontaneous animal tumors. Both in human tumors and in the spontaneous animal ones four mechanisms of angiogenic phenotype acquisition were identified. Avascular tumors recruit their own blood vessels. This is the most common mechanism of gaining an angiogenic phenotype.

About 95% of human malignant tumors are carcinomas that microscopically originate from in situ lesions, developed in the avascular epithelium, separated from the connective tissue's vascularization by the basal membrane. After neoangiogenesis stimulation by tumor cells, the basal membrane is not always immediately degraded. In mammary ductule and prostatic intraepithelial neoplasia, a ring formed of the new blood vessels arranged around the in situ lesion is observed. These vessels are temporarily separated from the tumor cells through the basal membrane. After its degradation, the new microvessels converge towards the tumor and are surrounded by malignant cells.

Circulating endothelial stem cells

Recently, circulating endothelial cells have been identified, apparently derived from the bone marrow. Such cells auto incorporate themselves in the microvessels of neovascularization areas. Once the area of neovascularization is initiated, endothelial cell precursors participate in the process of vascular development. It was shown that circulating endothelial cells can also be a target for therapy with angiostatin.

Stimulation of host cells

Some tumors stimulate the host's fibroblasts and attract them to the tumor site, in response to over expression of VEGF. Through this mechanism the already initiated angiogenic phenotype is amplified.

Cooption of vessels

In some metastasis, as observed in the cerebral metastasis, tumor cells leave the microvessels of the target organ and start to proliferate around them, causing apoptosis of pre-existing endothelial cells and ultimately induce the formation of vessel sprouts from the surrounding vessels. This process, called co-optation, may be an intermediate point or an alternative in winning the angiogenic phenotype.

Experiments on transgenic mice with spontaneous tumors suggest that only about 10% of tumor cells gain the angiogenic phenotype. The non-angiogenic cells are sustained by capillaries recruited by neighboring cells. Similarly, in human tumors areas with intense neovascularization and adjacent areas with a reduced number of blood vessels can be observed.

Significant progress has been made in terms of identifying the factors that control angiogenesis. It seems that endothelial growth factor VEGF has a central role, intervening both in the proliferation of endothelial cells and the formation of the vascular wall, both in physiological and pathological situations (Ferrara et al., 1999).

To date, five members of the VEGF family are known, alongside them others being recognized as important in the process of angiogenesis (Yancoupulos et al., 2000).

There are several known growth factors and cytokines, which naturally induce or promote angiogenesis by stimulating endothelial cell growth. The most important of these is VEGF initially known as the VEP, vascular permeability factor, due to its proven capability to increase vascular permeability. It has assigned a key role in tumor stroma formation (Devorak et al., 1993). VEGF is considered to be a stimulating factor for mitosis of endothelial cells (Connolly et al., 1989). It is considered that VEGF stimulates the whole cascade of processes involved in angiogenesis (Leung et al., 1989) and in addition substantially increases vascular permeability thus having a dual role in tumorigenesis. VEGF also functions as an apoptosis inhibitor for the endothelial cells of neoformation vessels (Benjamin et al., 1999). Several studies incriminate VEGF over expression in tumors of the breast, ovary, urinary bladder, uterus (Toi et al., 1999). In these cases the VEGF values are increased and blocking its activity with anti-VEGF or anti-VEGF receptor antibodies inhibits tumor growth (Kim K. et al., 1993). The therapeutic perspectives arose by these comments represent the objective of several experimental studies. From the therapeutic point of view both factors that stimulate angiogenesis, as well as those which inhibit it present interest. Those that stimulate the angiogenesis process are represented by the VEGF family, which alongside VEGF (VEGF-A), the most representative of them, further comprise: VEGF-B, VEGF-C, VEGF-D, VEGF-E (Yancoupoulos et al., 2000), platelet endothelial growth factor, angiopoietin1, angiopoietin 2 and the epinephrine family. Angiogenesis inhibitor factors are represented by a range of endogenous proteins, which could represent a starting point for anti-angiogenic therapy: alpha and beta interferon (Sinh et al., 1995), angiostatin, endostatin, vasostatin (Pike et al., 1998), antithrombin III (O'Reilly, et al. 1999). The angiogenesis process at the level of the tumor formations is schematically represented as follows: angiogenesis is mainly mediated by VEGF, which causes the proliferation of endothelial cells and the formation of vascular tubules. Under the action of angiopoietin 1 the maturation of neoformation vessels takes place. In the absence of VEGF the regression of this entire process occurs.There are several markers that may indicate the angiogenic activity in the tumor formations: CD31 and CD34 (Fay P. et al., 1993). Also anti-alpha smooth muscle actin antibodies from the smooth muscle fiber can make the difference between immature neoformation vessels and mature, well differentiated vessels from the tumor structure (Benjamin L. et al., 1999). The relationship between VEGF-mediated angiogenesis and ovarian tumor progression was demonstrated by several studies (Gordon et al., 1996). The presence of receptors for VEGF in ovarian tumors is correlated with a poor prognosis, suggesting that VEGF mediated angiogenesis stimulates disease progression (Boocock et al., 1995). So the angiogenesis process can be regarded as a prognostic factor in the evolution of ovarian tumors. An accurate indicator of angiogenic activity is represented by the microvascular density at the level of a tumor formation. An increased microvascular density is the result of an intense angiogenic activity and correlates with a poor prognosis (Y. Takahashi et al., 1995). Ovarian cancer is associated with large volumes of ascites. Starting from this fact the role of VEGF in the formation of ascites fluid in the ovarian hyperstimulation syndrome was investigated. Thus it was demonstrated that VEGF being a major hyperpermeability factor, it leads to the formation of ascites fluid in the aforementioned syndrome. The administration of anti-VEGF serum resulted in the reduction of ascites volume in 70% of cases (McClure et al., 1994). An attempt was made to establish the role of VEGF in the formation of ascites fluid in patients with ovarian cancer (Messiano et al., 1998). A model of in vivo ovarian cancer was developed by inoculation of an ovarian tumor cell line in mice, in which a previously state of immunosuppression had been induced. In one group the anti-VEGF monoclonal antibodies and VEGF receptor antagonists were administered (thereby neutralizing the activity of VEGF), after which the effects of blocking the activity of VEGF on tumor growth and formation of ascites fluid were tracked in comparison to the control group. During the administration of treatment tumor growth was significantly slowed down and ascites fluid production was completely inhibited. But after the discontinuation of treatment the disease advanced rapidly, with the development of ascites, cachexia and growth of the tumor formations. These observations outline the involvement of VEGF in tumor progression and ascites formation, opening at the meantime new therapeutic perspectives. Other studies have evaluated serum levels of VEGF in patients with cancer of the ovary, breast, colon or uterus. Serum levels were significantly increased in patients with ovarian cancer (Tempfer C. et al., 1998) in comparison to control group. Increased levels of VEGF were found in the fluid contained by of malignant ovarian cyst formations. The value of VEGF as a marker for tumor progression is discussed. Ovarian cancer, unlike other locations of the neoplastic disease, has peritoneal seeding as the primary means of dissemination, dissemination through the vascular mechanism being of reduced importance (Yang et al., 2006; Palmer et al., 2007). From this point of view the role of VEGF in ovarian cancer dissemination shifts to a secondary role.

The numerous and various substances with anti-angiogenic effect suggest that soon their indications and potential value in the treatment of cancer will be contoured. Although angiogenesis stimulated the enthusiasm of many researchers, there are a number of issues that limit the progress in this area. By their nature, many anti-angiogenic substances are difficult to assess in terms of their effectiveness in the early stages of clinical trials (Rossochacka-Rostalska et al., 2007). With only a few exceptions, anti-angiogenics do not determine a rapid regression of the tumor (in comparison with conventional cytotoxic agents). Thus, if a hemangioma or a giant tumor of the mandible is treated by chronic administration of interferon α2β no effects are seen for several months (Nilsson et al., 2005). After this period, the slow regression of these benign tumors follows. Due to these aspects, it becomes mandatory to rethink the models used and the testing of anti-angiogenics in several ways. It is likely the combined use of anti-angiogenic agent with conventional cytotoxic medication, some studies demonstrating a cumulative effect. Certainly, Herceptin increases the efficiency of chemotherapy in a certain proportion of advanced stages of breast cancer. Another possible solution to the problem may arise by improving the strategies based on antivascular targeted therapy, which cause acute tumor regression, as demonstrated in some experimental models. Such an effect is determined by Combretastin A-4, a substance that binds tubulin. This substance elicits an intravascular thrombogenic response, causing the degeneration of numerous endothelial cells, the collapse of the vascular network and death of numerous tumor cells (Mobasheri et al., 2005; Luo et al., 2005). Certainly drugs that have the ability to induce dramatic regression of the tumor without major toxic effects will be introduced (Penault-Llorca et al., 2003). Identification of molecular specific markers for endothelial cells of new formed blood vessels could form the basis for a more effective and safer therapy (Giatromanolaki et al., 2004; Beckers et al., 2005). In experimental situations, tumors can be excised and examined regarding blood supply, vascular structure, viability of endothelial cells and angiogenic activity markers. In clinical situations, serial biopsies of metastatic tumors are neither practical nor desirable. In these circumstances, it is required to identify "surrogate" angiogenic markers in serum or urine (currently no such marker exists, Taukagoshi et al., 2003). Nowadays, perhaps only the improvement of imaging methods can provide useful information regarding vascular structure and permeability (Cao et al., 2006; Rask et al., 2006; Mabuchi et al., 2007).

In conclusion, it can be stated that angiogenesis is an essential process for tumor growth and metastasis development, and VEGF, by its role in the angiogenesis process, is a key element in disease progression. These findings form the starting points for the development of new therapeutic strategies, in addition to those already elaborated, which unfortunately have shown their limitations.

Tumor lymphangiogenesis

Despite the clinical relevance, current knowledge on the vascular and lymphatic metastasis about is scant. The vast majority of studies in the last decade have focused on tumor angiogenesis, lymphangiogenesis being "forgotten" by most authors. The discovery and characterization of VEGF has brought up in concerns the lymphatic system, by the identification of VEGFR-3 in this family, which is predominantly expressed in the endothelial cells of lymphatic vessels and is an inhibitor of VEGF-C and D. Injected in transgenic mice it induces lymphatic vessel abnormalities in the dermis, but does not influence blood vessels. These results show that angiogenesis and lymphangiogenesis are controlled separately by different members of the VEGF family. Thus, the expression of VEGF-C induced using an insulin promoter in transgenic mice has demonstrated the formation of lymphatic vessels around the islets of Langerhans, which normally lack lymphatic vessels. The experiments that noted lymphatic vessels involution suggest that VEGF-C or its analogs could stimulate therapeutic lymphangiogenesis. Perhaps the most important observation relates to the fact that VEGF-C and D induce lymphangiogenesis and stimulate the production of lymphatic metastasis. It has been shown by using LYVE-1 antibody that the number of intra- and peritumoral lymphatic vessels is significantly higher in tumors overexpressing VEGF-C or D. Anti-VEGF-D antibodies significantly reduce the number of lymphatic metastases. Soluble VEGFR-3 inhibits tumor-associated lymphangiogenesis in human mammary carcinoma transplanted in mice. These experiments demonstrate that tumors can activate lymphangiogenesis, a neglected phenomenon until recently. Recent observations on lymphangiogenesis make this process occupy the central position in the research of cancer disease. Lymphangiogenesis has been more closely and more successfully studied only in the last decade, by the investigation of the prognostic role of lymphatic vascular density, as well as the clinical significance of growth factors and specific receptors involved in the process.

In ovarian tumors, the first articles published on the subject are recent (2000), probably due to the particular remote extension of this type of neoplasia (Sundar et al., 2006). Due to the uncertainties stated above, we have evaluated the clinical impact of lymphatic microvessel density in the last part of this study.

3. PECULIARITIES OF TUMOR VESSELS MORPHOLOGY IN OVARIAN CANCER

Ovarian malignant tumors have a great microscopical diversity, including: serous, mucinous, endometrioid, clear cell, sexual cords neoplasia etc, which require a relatively complicated classification, but essential in order to draw conclusions in the domain we have proposed. For this reason, in the first stage of our research we morphologically evaluated the peculiarities of vessels associated to tumors included in the study, although these issues do not bring relevant information to the angiogenesis process. For each of the cases we evaluated the structure of the tumor, the degree of differentiation, the particular aspects of normal limitrophe ovarian tissue as well as the variations of blood vessels in the tumor and peritumoral area detectable by this method. The incidence of various histopathological forms diagnosed was rendered in the previous chapter, and we did not considered appropriate to describe and exemplify them, since these aspect are well known from specialized treatises and the WHO classification of ovarian tumors. We considered all of this data is not mandatory to define the entities that we have investigated, from the point of view of angiogenesis and lymphangiogenesis in ovarian tumors.

On the other hand, the examination of preparations stained with conventional methods has been an important methodological component of our study, because it allowed the identification of peritumoral areas and areas of the tumor in which the maximum number of blood vessels was expected to be highlighted. For this purpose we have studied sections stained with hematoxylin-eosin and trichrome Masson methods.

The examination of normal ovarian tissue limitrophe to the tumor revealed the classical histological structures, with the presence of ovarian stroma and presence of corpus albicans. Given the age of the patients included in the study, we did not notice the presence of ovarian follicles except in two cases. Arteriolar type blood vessels showed a thick wall, and in the peripheral area of remaining medulla we identified very thin-walled blood vessels, occasionally containing red blood cells (Figure 1).

The structure and arrangement of blood vessels was significantly different in terms of morphology in the cases with ovarian carcinoma. When the tumor invaded the remaining medullar region in the form of isolated tumor isles, as shown in Figure 2a, the vessels did not have a different arrangement from the normal ones, except the fact that no small caliber vessels with a the tortuous course were identified.

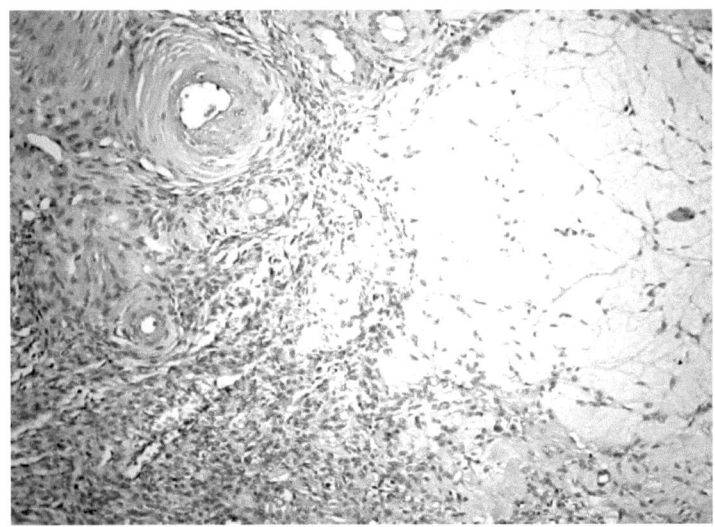
Figure 1. Blood vessels in a normal ovarian area. H&E stain, x100.

In diffuse proliferations, as we observed in the clear cell carcinoma, in the tumor stroma between the isles of malignant cells we noticed the exclusive presence of small caliber vessels with a very thin wall, located in the immediate vicinity of malignant cells (Figure 2b). A major prognostic factor is vascular invasion, which we noticed in 14 of the 62 patients included in the study (22.58%). The percentage is higher than that reported in literature, but on the other hand it was expected to be so, taking into consideration that most of the cases were classified as natural evolution stages III and IV at the moment of diagnosis.

Frequently, the tumor cells were present in the form of strings in small blood vessels (Figures 2c and d), nuclear pleomorphism being noticed even in these circumstances. The presence of massive emboli was less noticed, preferential in adenocarcinoma cases, in distended vessels, with a wide lumen, delimited by flattened endothelium (Figure 2e). Only in two of the serous adenocarcinoma cases we noticed the presence of tumor cells delimiting irregular spaces containing red blood cells, which indicates with the highest probability a particular form of angiogenesis, respectively vascular mimicry, and whose significance for the dissemination of ovarian tumors is not known until now.

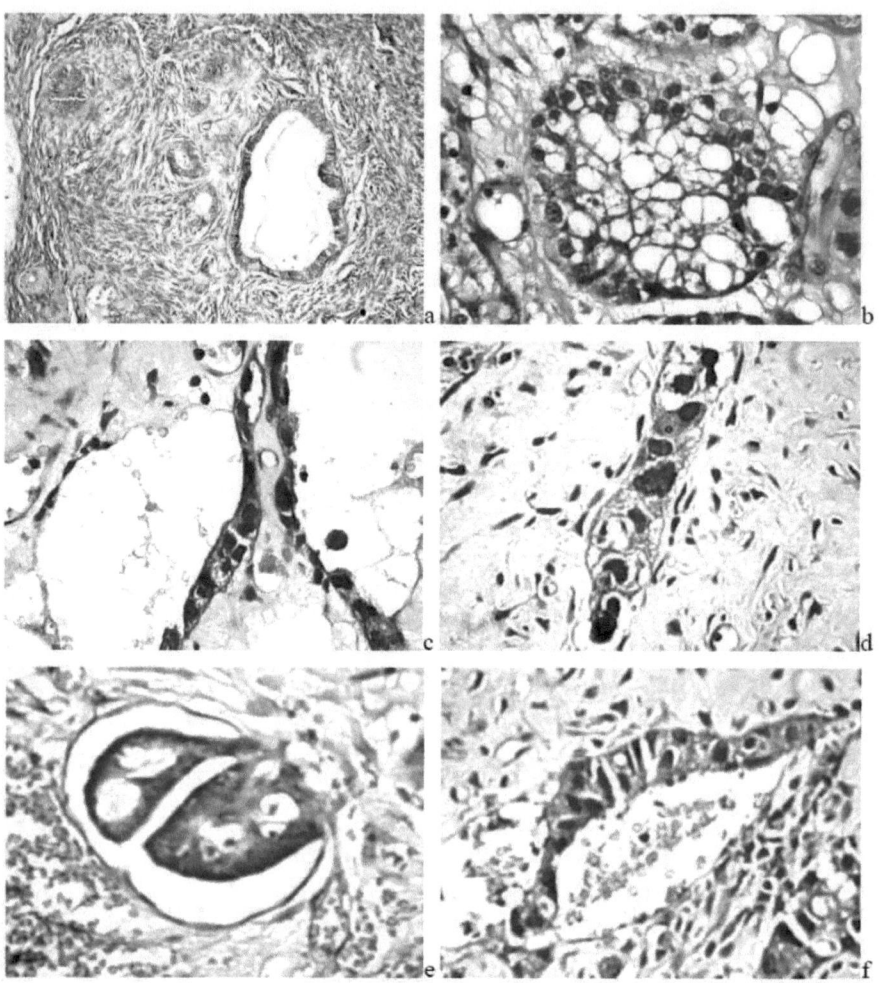

Figure 2. The particularities of the blood vessels associated with ovarian tumor
and the presence of invasion of blood vessels. Hematoxylin-eosin stain.

In the evaluation of these aspects we have not identified any peculiarities or
preferential disposition of blood vessels that can be correlated with the identified
histopathological forms, neither in any "classic" forms (id est serous, mucinous,
endometrioid, with clear cells or undifferentiated adenocarcinoma) nor in the
particular forms, as were Brenner, Sertoli or Leydig tumor (diagnosed in two cases,
one case and another case, respectively).

Most vessels identified on sections stained with conventional methods had a well defined wall with perivascular cells (Figure 3a). There were very few visible small vessels in the tumor area using morphological methods. At the invasion border broad vascular areas were identified, usually without content (Figure 3b). The vast majority of blood vessels in the endometrioid carcinomas (n = 6) were small in size, with a very thin, irregular and apparently discontinuous wall, with a distended lumen containing red blood cells (Figure 3c). Unlike these aspects, in the serous adenocarcinoma capillaries with a distinct regular and wall, arranged in a hyaline aspect mass, were present in the papillary axes (Figure 3d). The incompletely defined appearance of blood vessels was even more obvious in the clear cell carcinoma, where we frequently noticed wide lacunar spaces, with no content of figurative elements (Figures 3e and f).

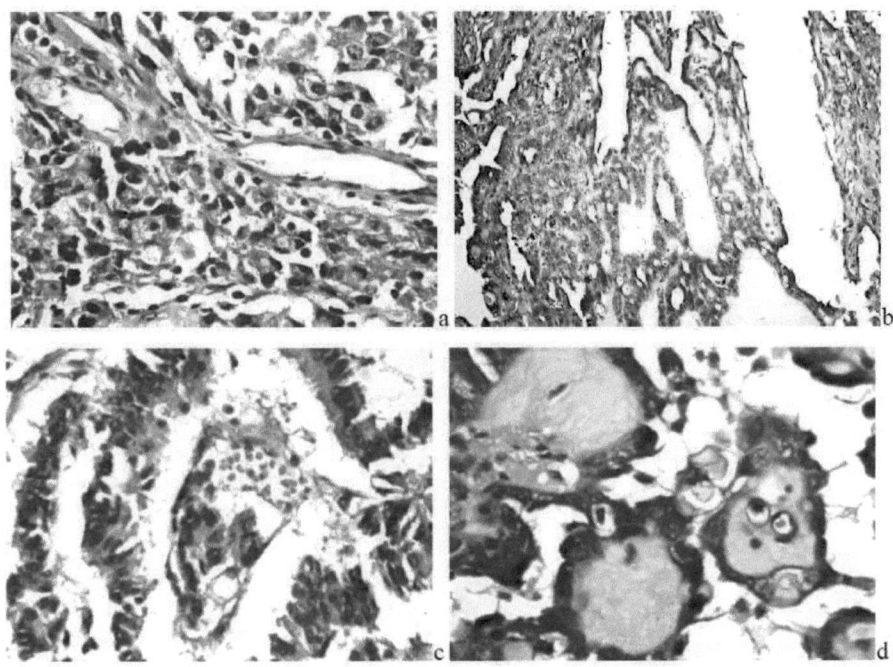

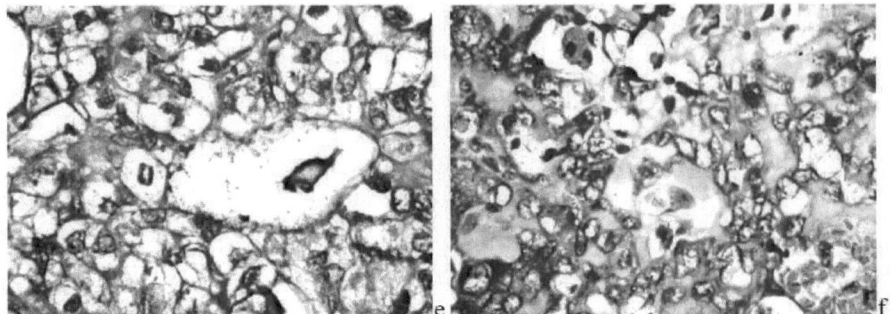

Figure 3. Ovarian tumor-associated blood vessels. Serous adenocarcinoma (a, b). Endometrioid (c). Serous (d). Clear cell (e and f).

The lowest number of blood vessels was noticed only in a single case of Sertoli cell tumor of this casuistry. The vessels were small in size, being located in the connective tissue between the areas of proliferating cells, whose architectural organization and acidophilic cytoplasm facilitated the diagnosis (Figure 4 a and b).

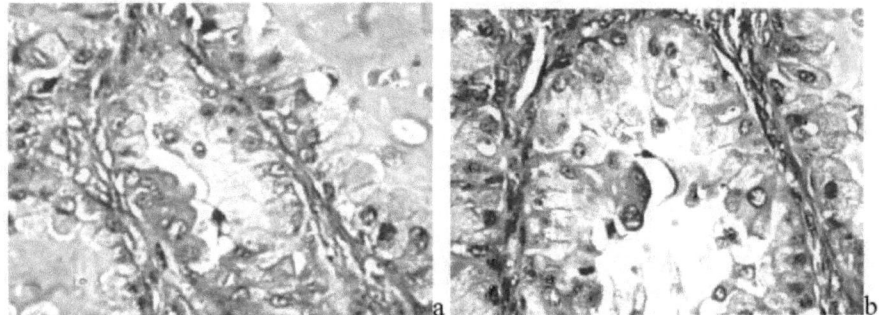

Figure 4. Sertoli cell tumor.

In the undifferentiated carcinoma, characterized by diffuse, infiltrative proliferation and tumor cells with severe anaplasia (Figure 5a and b), we did not identify with certainty the blood vessels on sections stained with the usual methods.

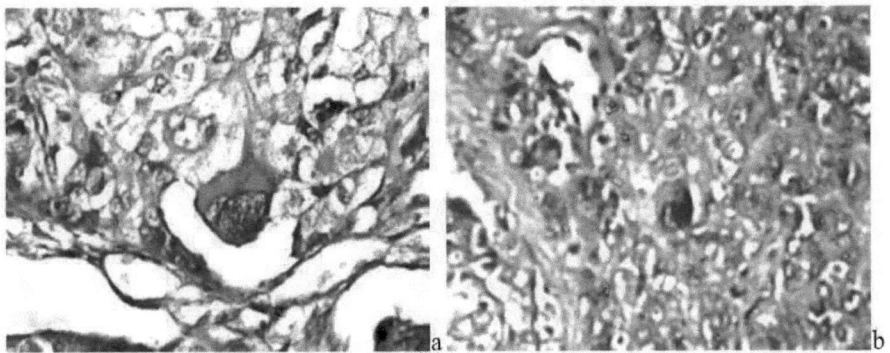

Figure 5. Undifferentiated carcinoma. In the tumor area one can not distinct elements suggestive of blood vessels.

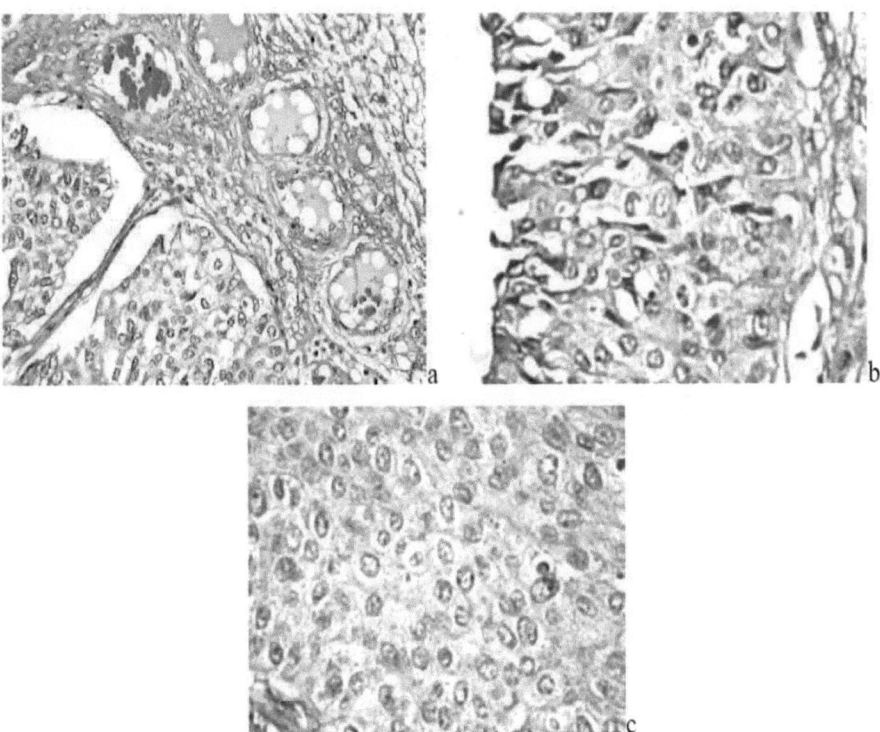

Figure 6. Brenner tumor with dilated peritumoral vessels and rare, very small, intratumoral vessels.

In the two Brenner tumor cases we noticed similar aspects in terms of vessel-arrangement and type of blood vessels. Thus, in the peritumoral area, the vessels were numerous, dilated, usually with aspects of stasis. In the tumor area the vessels were very rare, small in size, disposed between the tumor cells, and primarily recognized by the presence of red blood cells in the lumen (Figures 6 a, b, c).

In conclusion of this chapter, we state that morphological staining methods are less useful for identifying the type of ovarian tumor-associated blood vessels and have no predictive value for the angiogenic phenotype of the tumor. On the other hand they are useful in identifying the areas with high vascular density in tumor and peritumoral areas, as well as for the diagnosis of vascular invasion, which we identified in 22.58% of cases.

4. INTERPLAY BETWEEN ENDOTHELIAL AND PERIVASCULAR CELLS IN OVARIAN CANCER

The vessels from the tumoral and peritumoral aria of the ovarian neoplasia are structurally different from the vessels identified in the corresponding normal tissues. First of all, we identified significant numerical differences, translated through the values of the vascular microdensity. Secondly, we have noticed that the vessels associated to the neoplastic proliferation present irregular limits, a thin wall in the majority of cases, present a sinuous trajectory, and frequently, they present the tendency to form branches and anastomosis, thus giving birth to veritable networks located at the the borders and within the tumoral proliferation. On occasion, we have noticed the presence of peritumoral vascular proliferations mimicking the glomeruloid corpuscles. Throughout the years numerous trial have been carried out in order to classify tumour associated vessels on pure morphological bases, but none of these classifications as adopted, on one hand, because they did not offer any functional information, and on the other hand, due to the fact that perivascular cells, especially pericytes, proved to be difficult to identify at the time being, before applying immunohistochemistry on a large scale. Trials of this kind were recently applied in angiogenesis tumour studies. The associated tumour vessels were clasiffied as immature, intermediate and mature, based on the presence or absence of perfusion in case of the newly formed vessels, on the proliferative capacity of endothelial cells and on the presence or absence of perivascular cells. This methodology was applied in numerous consecutive studies made on a great variety of tumors and it has been demonstrated that in the tumoral and peritumoral aria, the number of immature and intermediate vessels is higher than the number of mature vessels, thus bringing new perspectives in that which considers antiangiogenic therapy (Cimpean and colab, 2005; Cimpean and colab, 2007).

Regarding this aspect, the scientific literature is lacking data in case of ovarian carcinomas and the normal ovary, despite the practical potential aspect, represented by the identification of the specific therapeutic vascular target. Due to these motives, we proposed to investigate the presence, distribution and incidence of these vessel types in both the tumoral and peritumoral aria by means of the double immunostaining method, based on the expression of a specific endothelial marker (CD34) and of smooth muscle actin (that evidences the presence of perivascular cells).

In order to realize the proposed objectives, we applied the immunostaining method based on the endothelial marker CD34 and the most specific marker of perivascular cells, that identifies the contractile filaments, namely smooth muscle actin. According to this working system, the final product of reaction for CD34 was stained in brown, and the pericyes/smooth muscle cells were stained in red. The quantification of the vessels identified according to the above mentioned classification, was based on the following criteria: the immature vessels were considered to be elements stained with CD34 only, without a visible lumen; the intermediate vessels presented a positive reaction for CD34 and an evident lumen, but did not present any perivascular cells; the mature vessels presented a lumen well lined by CD34 positive endothelial cells and perivascular cells. We used the marker CD34 due to its high sensibility, also based on the fact that there are no other positive cells in the stroma of ovarian carcinomas. The internal positive control of the double immunoreaction was represented by arteriolar pre-existing vessel types (fig. 7a) and by the venular ones (fig. 7b), in which case we have noticed a constant staining of the endothelial and perivascular components.

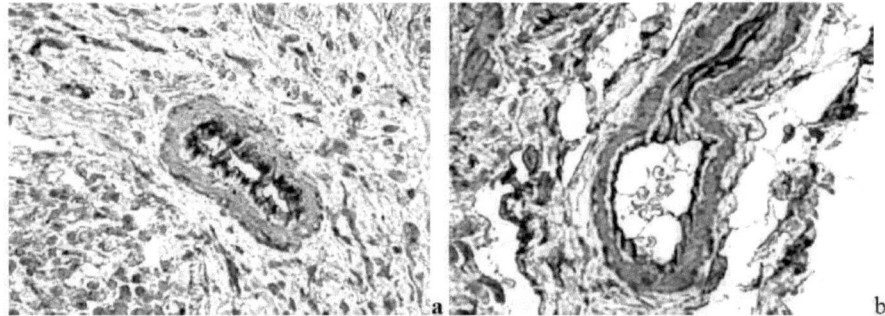

Figure 7. Double immunoreaction for CD34 (brown) and smooth muscle actin (red). The internal positive control on arteriolar vessels (a) and venular vessels (b).

All the three vessel types were observed in both the normal tissue located at a distance from the tumor proliferation, and in the peritumoral tissue, as well as in the tumoral area. Despite their presence, the proportion between the three vessel types was significantly different.

Therefore, in the normal tissue, over 80% of the vessels with lumen presented a distinct layer of perivascular cells, indicating the fact that the majority of these vessels are mature. This aspect was observed in both the medium size vessels as well as in case of the small vessels. The presence of blocked endothelial buds, positive for CD34, and assimilated with the immature type vessels, was considered to be determined by the remodelation of the vascular plexes from the ovarian stroma, but the percentage of 0.42% highlights the fact that at this age remodelation is minimum. The incidence of immature and intermediate vessels increases in the peritumoral tissue, with the persistence of the pre-existing mature vessels. Along with the mature vessels that have a well represented layer of perivascular cells, numerous vessels of small dimensions occur, these small vessels expressing only CD34 (fig. 8a). Also, transitional aspects may be observed on the short segments of the intermediate vessels walls, that express smooth muscle actin. In the peritumoral tissue the density of the immature, intermediate and partially mature vessels was significantly higher in the cases that presented a rich inflammatory infiltrate. In the tumor area, the immature and intermediate vessels were predominant. The immature vessels presented small dimensions, irregular shapes, no evident lumen, and were marked by chord cells that were positive only for CD34 (fig. 8b). We also identified intermediate vessels of large dimensions, with a large and irregular lumen, that express CD34 but not smooth muscle actin (fig. 8c). In the tumor area, the previously mentioned transitional aspects were significantly more frequent (fig. 8d). We observed the formation of irregular networks, with a focal disposition, that were composed of CD34 positive chords of cells, an aspect that suggests the rapid endothelial proliferation (fig. 8e).

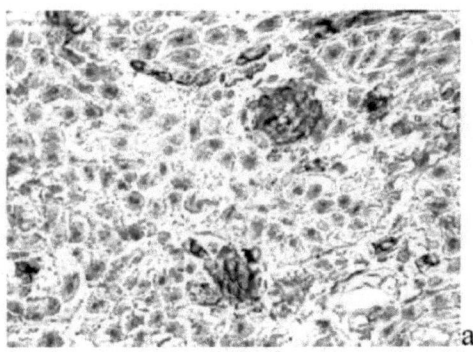

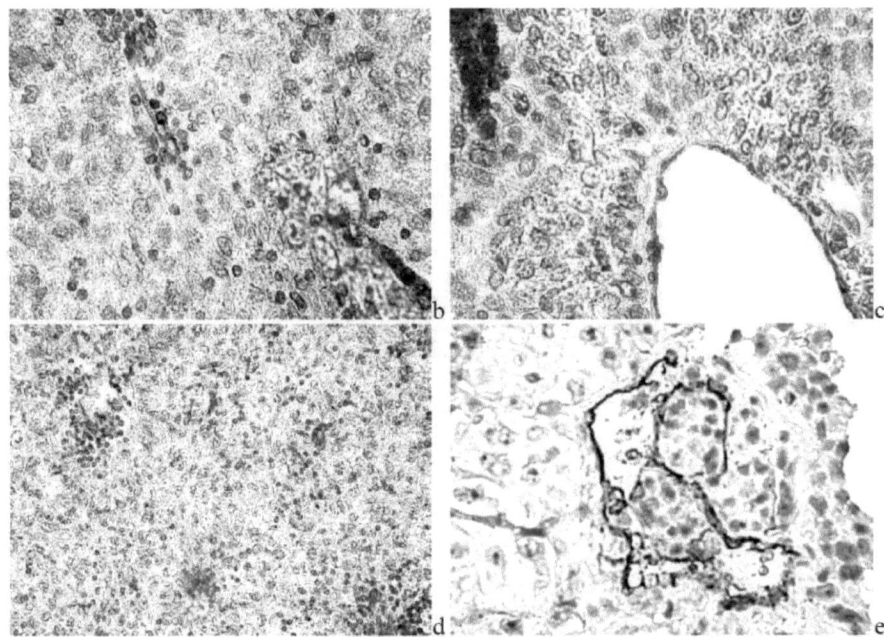

Figure 8. Mature, intermediate and immature vessels identified by means of
double immunoreaction for CD34 and smooth muscle actin.

The percentage values of the immature, intermediate and mature vessels in comparison to the total MVD, calculated in the previous chapter, though which it may be concluded that the mature vessels are predominant in the normal ovary, and immature vessels have been found to present low values. In ovarian carcinomas (serous, with clear cells, mucous and endometrioid) we have evaluated the tumoral and peritumoral areas and we have ob served that in the tumoral area, the majority of the vessels are of immature and intermediate type. We also observed high values for these parameters in the peritumoral area, but in this case, the pre-existing vessels that express actin are more numerous.

As particular aspects, we mention the two tumor types that we have included in this part of the study due to comparative reasons (Brenner and with Sertoli cells), in which case we observed a great number of mature vessels, while the immature ones were present only in the Brenner tumor having significantly lower values compared to the other vessel types.

Based on the obtained results after the evaluation of the blood vessels associated to the neoplastic ovarian proliferation using the method of double immunostaining with CD34/SMA, reveals the fact that in the normal tissue, the majority of the blood vessels are mature, and in the tumoral and peritumoral area, the majority of vessels are of immature and intermediate type. Based on the obtained results, unlike other authors, we consider that only the counting of immature and intermediate vessels may have a predictive value for the progression and metastasis and also, a predictive value for the response to antivascular therapy.

5. THE ACTIVATION AND PROLIFERATION RATE OF ENDOTHELIAL CELLS: A POTENTIAL MAKER OF THE RESPONSE TO ANTIANGIOGENIC THERAPY

The morphological character of the blood vessels, their type and MVD have been demonstrated as being prognostic factors in ovarian carcinomas. The progression of angiogenesis during the natural evolution of the neoplasia is realized through the sprouting and intususception phenomena as it has been demonstrated for the majority of human solid tumors and in different experimental models. The signalizing pathways that induce the formation of new blood vessels are already quite well known, but surprisingly, the target of these signals, the responding endothelial cells respectively, is scarcely characterized. Therefore, it is not yet known which are the endothelial cells that commence the sprouting process, the division and the migration, and the means through which they are activated. Due to these uncertainties, numerous authors attempted to identify a marker with a high specificity for the activated endothelial cells, and until now, the most known marker from this cathgory is CD105, also known as endogline.

Although there is no strictly specific marker for the tumor vasculature, nowadays, a few candidates with potential therapeutic implications are known. One of the most promising is endogline, CD105, preferentially expressed in the angiogenic endothelial cells. This property represented the motive for which CD105 was identified as a primary target for tumor imaging, prognosis and therapy. Endoglin is expressed at the cell surface as a 180 kDa homoldymeric transmembranar protein.

The external domain links TGF beta 1, and the gene that encodes it is located on chromosome 9q34. Until now, two isoforms with a different number of amino acid residues have been identified. The main source for endogline is represented by the endothelial cells, and it is intensely expressed especially in the umbilical chord.

High levels have been observed in the sincytotrophoblast from the mature placenta and low quantities have been noticed in the vascular smooth muscle cells, fibroblasts, macrophages, eritroid precursors and pre-B leukemia cells.

Although the mechanisms of endogline actions and its functions are not fully characterized, it has been observed that in case of Knock-out CD105 mice multiple cardiovascular anomalies occur, thus determining their deaths in early embryonic stage.

The absence of CD105 restricts maturation and remodeling of blood vessels, determining dilations and ruptures of the vessels. CD105 exhibits a high specificity for the tumor vasculature in comparison to panendothelial markers.

Vascular microdensity calculated on specimens stained for endogline determination are correlated with breast cancer survival rate, unlike the method based on CD34 determination. Similar to prostate cancer, engogline expression was correlated with its stage, the Gleason score, metastases, the proliferation and survival index.

These correlations were not observed on specimens stained for the von Willebrand factor. Autoradiographic and immunohistochemical studies demonstrated that CD105 accumulates at the tumor periphery, where the maximum density of blood vessels is found, and the center of the tumor was hetherogenously stained. From all of these points of view, CD105 represents the ideal therapeutic target, due to the fact that specific antibodies do not react with normal endothelial cells. Despite this fact, the problem appears to be a bit more complicated, because endogline expression in the normal tissues is not completely known and also, some tumor cells present a cytoplasmic pattern of endogline expression, with no explanation of this phenomenon what so ever. On the other hand, MVD calculated using any staining based on an endothelial marker, although having prognostic value, does not represent a criteria for estimating the antiangiogenic therapeutic response.

At the time being, it is considered that the endothelial cells proliferation index is one of the few morphological methods with a predictive value from this point of view. Ki67 is a marker of cell proliferation (Scholzen and Gerdes 2000), that defines proliferation in both tumor cells and endothelial cells. During the interphase, antigen ki-67 may be exclusively detected in the nucleus, and during mitosis, the protein is restricted to the surface of the chromosomes. Ki-67 is present in all the active phases of the cell cycle (G1, S, G2, and mitosis), but it is not expressed by dormant cells (G0).

Numerous literature data associate endogline expression with the high proliferation rate of endothelial cells in vitro (Lebrin et al, 2004). Due to these motives, we investigated endogline and ki-67 expressions on the cases included in the study, in order to evaluate the succession of events regarding endothelial cells activation and proliferation from the tumoral and peritumoral areas. In order to evaluate endothelial cells activation and proliferation we made use of the immunohistochemical method for CD105 and the double immunoreactions for CD34 and Ki67. We considered only the cells that express the two markers in our evaluation, in order to avoid confusion with tumor cells, that may also express Ki67.

In case of endogline reaction we observed the predominance of positive vessels in the tumor area and at the border between the tumor cells and the stroma. All the endogline positive vessels had small dimensions, an irregular contour, frequently presenting a septated lumen (fig.9a). Their number was greater, but statistically insignificant, in the areas presenting inflammatory infiltrate (fig. 9b). MVD calculated for CD105 was significantly greater in case of low differentiated tumors (fig. 9c), and in these cases, the newly formed vessels were constituted proper plexi that occasionally made the counting process very difficult (fig. 9d). On all sections, the medium values for MVD from the tumor area were 23.44, unlike the peritumoral area, for which only 14.33 of vessels were stained for this marker (fig. 9e and f). Constantly, the vessels that expressed CD105 did not present any positive endothelial cells for KI-67, thus signalizing the fact that activation and proliferation are distinct phases in the development of the vascular network in ovarian tumors.

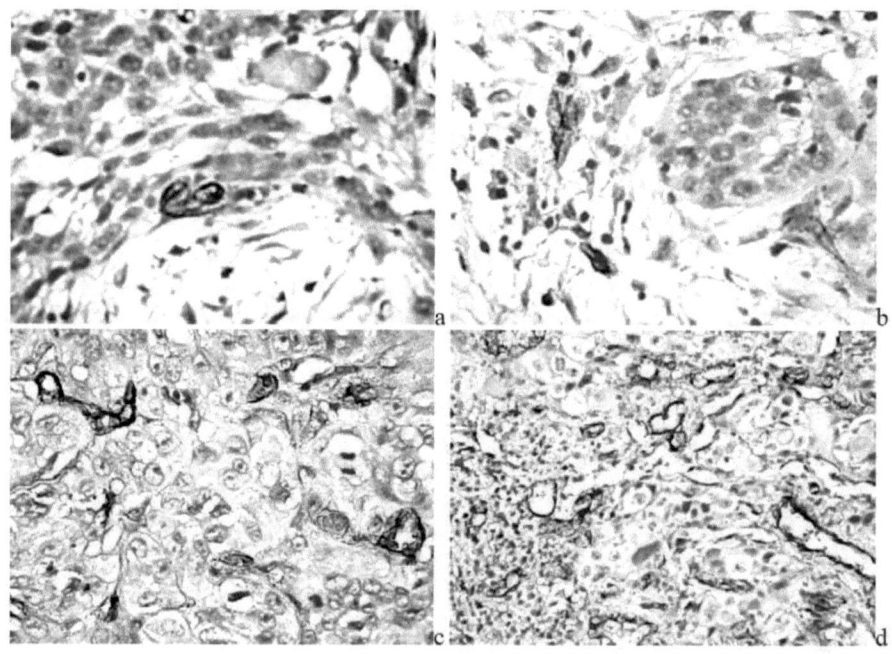

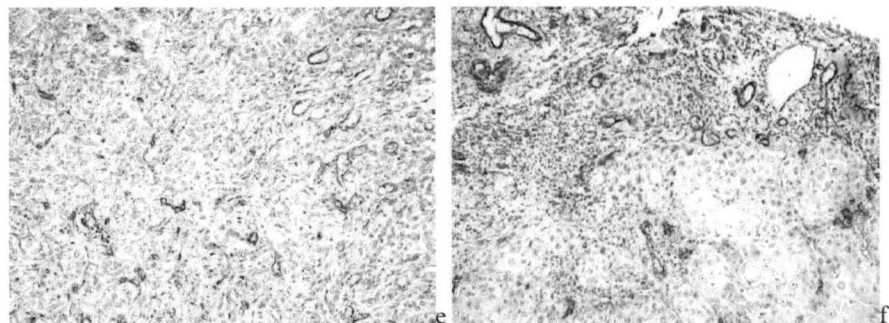

Figure 9. Endogline expression in ovarian tumors. Small irregular vessels (a), multiple in the tumor area (b), numerous in the non-differentiated carcinoma (c), forming intratumoral vascular plexi (d). The difference between the tumoral and peritumoral area (e and f). CD105 immunoreaction.

The immunohistochemical reaction for Ki-67 as the unique method, pointed out the presence of the final product of reaction in the tumor and stromal cells, including those from the vascular wall. In case of mature vessels from the stroma, we rarely observed the presence of positive perivascular cells (fig. 10a) and more frequently the presence of endothelial cells with intensely stained nuclei (fig. 10b). In the peritumoral zone, the evaluation of endothelial cells proliferation rate proved to be relatively easy, only the incidence of positive cells that line the vascular lumen being evaluated and the positive reaction rate was 4.5%. Unlike the peritumoral zone, at the tumor-stroma interface and in the middle of the tumor area, the evaluation of the endothelial cells proliferation rate was not possible by using only one antibody, because the majority of tumor cells were also positive (fig. 10c and d). Under these circumstances we made use of the double immunoreactions for Ki-67 and CD34 (fig. 11).

By using this method we observed the existence of a correlation between the vessel types and the presence of KI-67 positive endothelial cells in the tumor area. Therefore, in case of the vessels exhibiting a relatively large, irregular lumen, the endothelial cells were negative for KI-67 (fig. 12a), with rare exceptions, a it is observed in fig. 12b. The majority of masses from the peritumoral zone were positive for CD34, but negative for Ki-67, pointing out a very low endothelial cells proliferation rate (fig. 12c-e). This aspect was constant, independent from vessel dimension and morphology. In the tumor area, in case of numerous vessels located amongst neoplastic cells we noticed CD34 and Ki-67 co-expression, the proliferation rate for endothelial cells being estimated at 11.2% (fig. 12f).

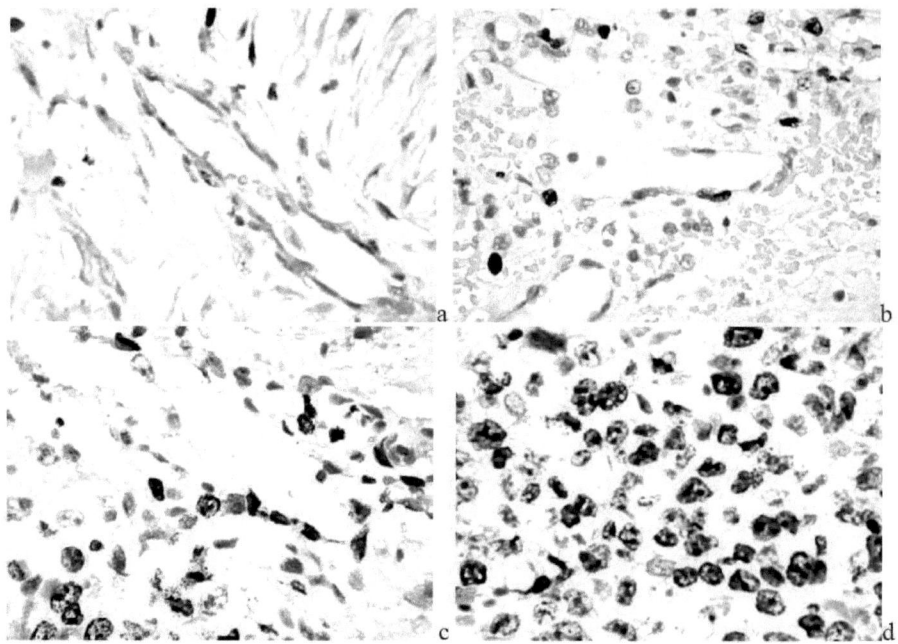

Figure 10. KI67 expression in ovarian tumors. The peritumoral tissue (a and b). The intratumoral area, with numerous positive malignant cells (c and d).

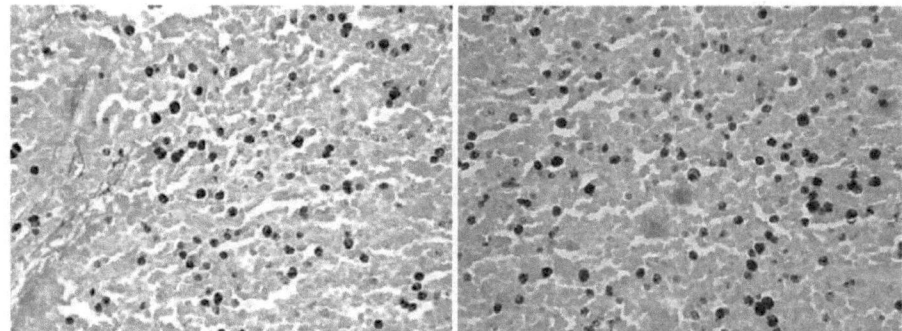

Figure 11. Double immunoreaction for Ki67 and CD34.

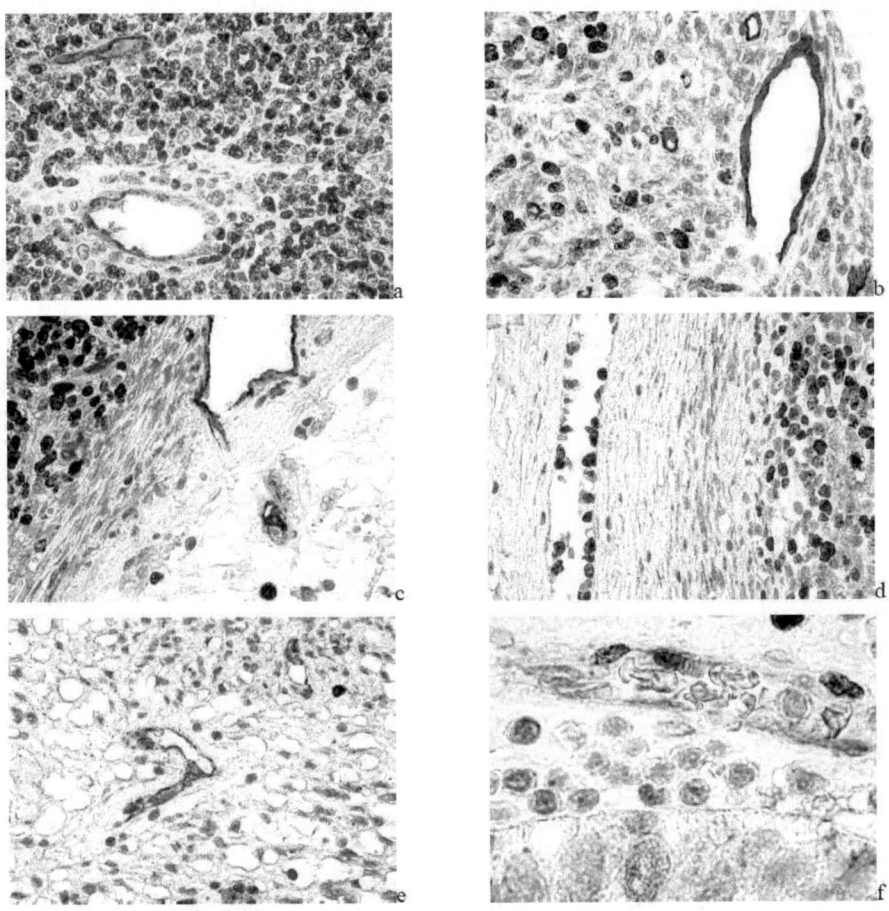

Figure 12. Double immunoreactions for KI67 (brown)/CD34 (red) (a-f).

Based on the obtained results, we believe that the activation of endothelial cells represents a distinct phase in ovarian tumor associated angiogenesis and that the majority of CD105 positive vessels are located in the tumor area. MVD calculated for the tumor and peritumor areas supports this statement, and the KI67 positive endothelial cells were not observed in case of CD105 positive vessels. The proliferation rate of endothelial cells from the vessels belonging to the tumor area is 11.2%, unlike the peritumoral blood vessels, characterized by an endothelial proliferation of 4.5%. Based on these results, we consider that the activation and proliferation of endothelial cells are distinct markers of tumor angiogenesis in ovarian cancer and their evaluation may be useful for monitoring the antiangiogenic and/or antivascular therapeutic response.

Ovarian cancer is the main cause of death amongst malignant gynecological lesions in developed countries and the majority of female patients are first diagnosed in advanced stages of the natural evolution of the disease. Numerous female patients are diagnosed in the peritoneal dissemination stage as it results from our statistics, and unfortunately, this type of dissemination does not present any clinically significant symptomatology. The high incidence of this neoplastic affection (reported at 13.9%000 by the USA National Cancer Institute) associated with a specific mortality rate of 8.9%000, signalizes the necessity of extensive studies regarding ovarian tumors behavior and molecular profile, as well as the urgent identification of new therapeutic targets. Despite the remarkable progresses in the last decades in the field of early cancer depiction and adjuvant therapy, the survival rate of female patients with ovarian cancer remains at low values, only 53% after 5 years of surveillance, no matter the present adjuvant therapy.

More than half of the ovarian tumors occur from the covering epithelium, from the mezothelial tissue, that presents a multipotent character and may differentiate itself in various other epithelial types (including endometrial, tubar, mucinous, urothelial). The particularities of distribution for the histopathological forms were also identified in the present study. However, the histogenesis of ovarian tumors is not yet elucidated, the models at hand being incomplete hypotheses sustained by proofs (Nisolle and co., 2007).

The variability of the total survival and the response to chemotherapy in case of female patients with ovarian cancer is significantly different, even if they are included in the same FIGO stage, histopathological type, differentiation grade or age group. The clinical results obtained through the treatment of human malignant tumors demonstrated that this variability is determined on one hand and generated by the unpredictable behavior of tumor cells, by the cytokines effects secreted by them, but on the other hand it is determined by the tumor microenvironment, that includes angiogenesis and lymphangiogenesis. Due to these motives, the report not only of classic pathologic factors (that include the histopathological type and grade), but also the detected molecular anomalies comes as a stringent necessity for undergoing individualized therapy though targeted and individualized means.

The normal ovary is frequently used as an example for postnatal life angiogenesis. In the female reproductive system the formation and cyclic regression of blood vessels, a phenomenon orchestrated by the hormone stimuli, are evident. The development of ovarian follicles is accompanied by cell-tissue modifications, remodeling and fluid accumulation, and the intervention of VEGF in these stages, through its hiperpervious action. After ovulation the development of a rich vasculature that may be observed especially in the lutheal body appears a necessity. The normal vasculature development also contributes to steroid transportation at the action site, after which it dramatically regresses before the next cycle occurs. Although the factors that select the dominant ovarian follicle are too little known, around it, a significantly larger number of vessels have been observed than around those that will degenerate through athresia. A vasculature wave commences in the external sheath and the number of vessels increases along with the increase in the number of ganulosal cell rows. It is possible that this effect to be due to the growth factor gradient. In the secondary ovarian follicle a high rate of endothelial cells proliferation has been demonstrated (24-30%) through bromodeoxyuridine incorporation in CD31 positive cells and the dramatically increases up to 80% in the lutheal body. Endothelial proliferation is reduced in the middle f the lutheal phase, and lutheal regression coincides with the regression of the vessels.

Amongst the mechanism that contribute to the development of tumor angiogenesis, cooptation of host vessels is predominant in ovarian cancer, as it is observed in primary tumors restricted to the ovary, but also in case of peritoneal metastases. In this ultimate situation, tumor cells adhere to the mezothelial peritoneum from the immediate vicinity of some pre-existing blood vessels. Peritoneal dissemination is followed by the synthesis of growth factors in the moment in which the metastases reach their critical mass and hypoxia occurs, being followed by the formation of new blood vessels. This is not the only mechanism for the development of associated ovarian tumor vessels, but on the other hand, there are no data regarding the endothelial insertion of progenitor cells of medullar origin at the time being.

The prognostic impact of angiogenesis on the prognosis of female patients with ovarian cancer was studied by more than one group of authors. These studies were made in order to characterize new predictive elements for the unfavorable prognosis and consecutively, in order to include these female patients in the modern accepted therapies based on antiangiogenic medication, that may significantly increase their survival rate, as adjuvant therapy.

One of the parameters that in a way reflects malignant tumors angiogenesis is the microvascular density (MVD). In some moments of evolution for this concept, MVD was the only means to estimate the tumors angiogenic potential, and due to this aspect, at the time being, thousands of articles focused on this subject, concerning almost human tumor types are available (Gadducci and co., 2006). Following the enthusiasm initiated by this method, nowadays, not only its values but also its limits are known. The data regarding ovarian tumors associated MVD are controversial and this represents the main reason for which we have approached this subject during our study.

MVD estimation was filled with subjectivism for a long time, a subjectivism that was generated by the methods used for the counting process. MVD evaluated by using computerized systems of microscopic image analysis is correlated with the general survival of individual female patients and, as expected, it is not correlated with the age of the investigated female patients (Raspollini and co., 2005). Previous studies on ovarian cancer have shown that the quantity of residual tumor tissue is an important prognostic factor. In some series of female patients these elements had no statistical relevance, possibly due to the minimum quantity of residual tumor tissue. In the evaluation of ovarian tumors angiogenesis based on MVD estimation, we observed a statistically significant inversed correlation between this parameter and trombospondine-1 expression. Similar data have also been reported by other authors for trombospondine-2 also in ovarian cancer, thus turning this family of substances into potential contributors to complex antivascular therapy (Czekierdowski and co., 2008).

Microvascular density, investigated by a great number of authors, is considered an important prognostic factor in ovarian carcinomas, as well as in other human malignant tumors (Weidner et al, 1992; Eccles and co., 2008). The results of the correlations between MVD and prognosis were usually controversial in case of the same tumor type. We consider that the differences result especially from the process of counting all the marked vessels by using a specific endothelial antigen and with the highest probability, superior results from this point of view are obtained though counting the immature and mature vessels only. Moreover, we have also taken into consideration when counting MVD the immature, non-perfused vessels, an aspect that is excluded by a great number of authors, but accepted and carried out by others (Duff and co, 2003; Amis and co., 2005). Due to these motives, it is considered that MVD evaluation based on a marker of endothelial cell activation may be superior from a prognostic point of view (Minhajat et al., 2006).

Between the normal and intratumoral blood vessels there are a series of major differences. Intratumoral vessels often have an incompletely maturated wall and as a consequence, the architecture is abnormal. The collapse of intratumoral vessels is frequent, generating hypoxia followed by necrosis and under these circumstances, they are no longer able to support the rapid growth of tumor cells. Tumor vessels specifically express endogline (CD105), a homodimeric component on the surface of the TGFbeta receptor. Endogline is intensely expressed ny endothelial cells belonging to the intratumoral vessels, but not by the pre-existing blood vessels. Due to this motiv, the anti-CD105 antibody is useful for the differentiation between the normal vessels and those formed through tumor angiogenesis. Our results support this statement, through the fact that the majority of vessels from the tumor area were Cd105 positive, with an irregular aspect, unlike those from the peritumoral area in which the majority of vessels were negative. Our data confirm those from the literature, Taskiran and co (2006) identifying CD105 as an independent prognostic factor.

Tumor vessels may be segregated in three categories, based on their dimensions, perfusion, proliferation of endothelial cells and the presence of pericytes: perfused endothelial cell buds, intermediate and mature.

The immature vessels constituted of endothelial cell buds that emerge from the wall of functional vessels, are not perfused and have shown a high proliferation rate. The buds may be represented by isolated endothelial cells, without a visible lumen, positive for CD31 and von Willebrand factor. These cells are negative for protein S100 and represent between 18 and 25% of the total number of intratumoral vascular structures in case of large tumors and are predominant from a numerical point of view in case of small-size tumors. Isolated endothelial cells are not perfused and are not stained with Hoechst 33342 reagent that makes the nuclei of endothelial cells exposed to the blood flow. The proliferation rate demonstrated by using PCNA ranges between 39 and 69%.

The intermediate vessels are small, patent, and do not present in the constitution of their wall pericytes or smooth muscle cells. They are perfused vessels, in which over 90% of the endothelial cells are stained with Hoechst 33342 reagent. The incidence of this type of intratumoral vessels ranges between 33 and 43%.

The mature vessels are big, with a large lumen and a thin wall, the endothelial cells are in a dormant stage, presenting a minimum proliferative potential, their wall contains pericytes and they rarely form endothelial buds. The proliferation rate is low, the PCNA index ranging between 12 and 18% (Cohen, 1996). These vessels repetitively branch themselves and give birth to the intermediate ones that lack pericytes (Schoenfeld and co., 1994; Wu and co., 1994; Okamura and co., 1995).

The three types of intratumoral vessels may be evidenced by using the double immunostaining for CD31 (or CD34) and smooth muscle actin, the last being positive for both the smooth muscle cells from the vessel wall and pericytes. The majority of vessels from growing tumors are immature and intermediate. Antiangiogenic therapy drastically reduced the number of these vessels, while the mature ones do not present any significant numeric changes. The grade of maturation for newly formed vessels is correlated with the response to the therapy based on inhibitors of angiogenesis (Pan and co., 2008; Labiche and co., 2009; Rubatt and co., 2009). The classification of intratumoral vessels in these categories signalizes the fact that the therapeutic target is represented by immature and intermediate vessels, an aspect that has also been experimentally demonstrated on animals with interleukin-12 treated tumors. These observations have generated a new individualized antivascular therapeutic strategy targeted on pericytes (Lu and co., 2007; Lu and co., 2010).

Our results are according to those published by other authors regarding prostate cancer (Wilkstrom et al., 2002; Mok and co., 2009). These authors have identified only 19% mature vessels in the tumor area, the majority being immature and intermediate. We mention that from the data that were available to us, we did not identify other studies that investigated the morphological character of the vessels from the tumor area in ovarian carcinomas in this manner. These aspects may be correlated with the modulation of the angiogenic phenotype, as it has been demonstrated in an experimental model of ovarian epithelial cells (Goodheart and co., 2005; Schumacher and co., 2007; Chuck and co., 2010).

The introduction of taxol and cisplatin in ovarian cancer therapy has increased the survival rate (Rosano and co., 2010; Ghosh and co., 2010). Despite these prognostic benefits, only few female patients manage to survive a la long, and the development of some primary more efficient therapies remains a necessity. Female patients with ovarian cancer resistant to cisplatin therapy who do not respond to targeted therapy or present short term recurrence since the commencing the therapy continue to represent a difficult problem to solve (Polcher and co., 2010; Merritt and co., 2010; Darcy and Birrer, 2010). Tumor growth highly depends on the vasculature, and the aggressiveness is conferred, at least partially, by the microvascular density. As a consequence, the characterization of the angiogenic phenotype in case of ovarian tumors is essential for the prognosis and therapeutic strategy.

Chemotheray has effects on both tumor cells and on blood vessels (Chiyoda and co., 2010; KaKu and co., 2010). Paclitaxel in particular exhibits an antiangiogenic activity at subtoxic concentrations through inhibiting endothelial cell migration (Kim and co., 2007; Ghaemmaghami and co., 2010). Due to this motive, new antiangiogenic drugs with low toxicity from the taxan family are in the phase of clinical trial. Metronomically administrated chemotherapy significantly increases the efficiency of antiangiogenic therapy in ovarian cancer (Kamat and co., 2007; Lin and co., 2007).

At the time being, we do not dispose of certain data regarding the angiogenic changes of ovarian tumor under the influence of chemotherapy, although numerous studies have been carried out on the matter (Hata and co., 2004; Hata and co., 1998).

In the present study we have shown that the progenitor endothelial cell markers, AC133 and Tie2 are suppressed in the ovarian tumor vessels and in case of a limited number of tumor, and in malignant cells. EPCs are characterized by the coexpression of the two markers to which Cd=D34 and VEGFR2 are associated. Tie2 expression was signalized by other authors as well, but they did not correlate the reaction model with VEGF expression (Hata and co., 2004). Starting from the data that were available to us, we did not identify another study that signalized the presence of AC133 positive endothelial cells in case of female patients with ovarian cancer.

6. ENDOTHELIAL PROGENITOR CELLS

It is well known that the growth of new blood vessels is a component of certain pathological conditions, including tumor growth and metastasis. Previous experimental studies have suggested that bone marrow(BM)-derived circulating endothelial progenitor cells (EPCs) migrate to neovascularization sites and differentiate into endothelial cells in situ, a process termed vasculogenesis (Qin Ha and co., 2014; Tai Sun and co., 2012). Endothelial progenitor cells (EPCs) are bone marrow-derived cells that can be found in peripheral and umbilical cord blood. Recently, increasing amounts of data have revealed that bone-marrow (BM)-derived EPCs can foster the initiation and maintenance of angiogenic processes by integrating into developing vasculature under hypoxic conditions and into tumors. EPCs possess a high proliferation potential and have been found to be a potential marker for both neovascularization and response to antiangiogenic therapies (Qin Ha and co., 2014, Kawamoto and co., 2007).The cells were first isolated in the study by Asahara et al (1997), where it was demonstrated that cluster of differentiation 34-positive (CD34+) hematopoietic progenitor cells from adults can differentiate ex vivo into the endothelial phenotype (Qin Ha and co., 2014). These cells express endothelial markers and are incorporated into the neoformation vessels in ischemic areas. Data in the literature have supported the presence of circulating hemangioblasts in adults, and EPCs are defined as CD34- and VEGFR2-expressing elements (Tai Sun and co., 2012, Kawamoto and co., 2007). CD133, also known as prominin or AC133, is a conserved antigen with unknown biological activity, which is expressed by hematopoietic stem cells, but is absent in mature endothelial cells and in the monocyte line (Asahara and co., 1997). Under these conditions, CD133+/VEGFR2+ cells are likely to reflect immature progenitors and the cells interspersed in the vascular endothelium. Santarelli et al used mouse tumor models to demonstrate that BM-derived EPCs are greatly mobilized into the bloodstream, and home specifically to tumor tissues. In the tumor microenvironment, the recruited EPCs merged with the walls of a growing blood vessel, where they differentiated into endothelial cells and so promoted tumor growth. It has been reported that, during cancer proliferation, the number of circulating BM- derived progenitor cells increases dramatically. Circulating BM-derived EPCs have been used to determine the optimal dose of antiangiogenic drugs, most successfully in breast cancer (Peichev and co., 2000). In addition, Taylor proved that high levels of circulating BM-derived progenitor cells are correlated with tumor metastatic status. Recently, the contribution of EPCs to tumor angiogenesis has also been reported in clinical tumor samples from 6 patients who received bone marrow transplants from donors of the opposite sex. The endothelial cells within the tumor vessels were of donor origin, as shown by the mismatched sex chromosomes (Shi Q. and co., 1998). EPCs are considered bone-marrow derived cells that migrate into the peripheral blood in response to cytokines such as VEGF (Grigoras and co., 2014). In contrast to the ischemic condition, the role of circulating EPCs in tumor angiogenesis and growth is unclear. EPCs possess a high proliferation potential and have been found to be a potential marker for both neovascularization and response to antiangiogenic therapies (Santarelli and co., 2006). The role EPCs in cancer angiogenesis and growth deserves further investigation, especially in regard to their potential as markers to monitor disease progression or treatment response. In the group of circulating blood mononuclear cells there may be several sources of EPCs, including hematopoietic stem cells, myeloid cells that can differentiate on endothelial cells by growing, other progenitor circulating cells and mature endothelial circulating cells. The first evidence of the existence of several circulating EPCs was reported by Lin et al. Although the existence of EPCs has been demonstrated, with regard to malignant tumors the data is controversial on the pre-existing endothelium insertion rate and the extent to which these cells contribute to tumor angiogenesis. From these points of view, the results obtained so far vary between the extremely wide limits of 0 and 72 % for various human tumors. At present, the significance of circulating EPCs and the contribution of EPCs to tumor vessels have been confirmed in only a few solid malignancies, such as malignant glioma (Shi Q. and co., 1998), lung cancer (Fürstenberger and co., 2006), and mammal tumors (Peters and co., 2005). Increased levels of EPCs in peripheral blood were identified in patients with pancreatic carcinoma (Asahara and co., 1997), ovarian cancer (Shi Q. and co., 1998), non-small cell lung (Grigoras and co., 2014) and gastric (Santarelli and co., 2006) cancer. Consequently, the level of EPCs has been proposed as a novel biomarker for the diagnosis and monitoring of these lesions. However, the extent to which EPCs contribute to the generation of the tumor vessels varies significantly across different studies, from substantial to zero (Li B and co, 2006; Yajuan and co., 2010). The role of EPCs in neovascularization has been the subject of great debate. The quantity and clinical relevance of circulating endothelial progenitor cells in human ovarian cancer has been investigated by Sun and co. A relationship between circulating levels of EPC and the stage of the disease has been found, the circulating EPCs levels in the peripheral blood of stage III and IV ovarian cancer patients being significantly higher than that of stage I and II patients. The relationship between treatment type and EPCs levels has also been determined and moreover, surgery and chemotherapy significantly reduced the number of EPCs per ml of peripheral blood. However, after treatment, EPCs levels in the patients who underwent surgery and in the patients who received chemotherapy treatment were still elevated compared with healthy controls. It seems that circulating EPCs may have potential as a biomarker for monitoring tumor progression and angiogenesis. With the advent of molecular-targeted therapies, treatment for ovarian cancer is now moving beyond conventional chemotherapy. Inhibition of the specific cytokines essential for tumor vascularization is one such a therapy (Tai Sun and co., 2012); thus, anti-angiogenesis therapy has become a new strategy for ovarian cancer treatment. No proven bio-markers of tumor angiogenesis have been fully characterized; however, tumor microvascular density is used to predict tumor metastasis, recurrence, and prognosis.(Tai Sun and co., 2012; Yajuan and co., 2010). So far, no such studies have reported the contribution of EPCs in ovarian tumors. For this reason, the present study evaluated the expression of two markers, AC133 and tyrosine kinase with immunoglobulin-like and EGF-like domains 2 (Tie2), which signal the presence of EPCs in the pre-existing endothelium. In the group of circulating blood mononuclear cells there may be several sources of EPCs, including hematopoietic stem cells, myeloid cells that can differentiate on endothelial cells by growing, other progenitor circulating cells and mature endothelial circulating cells. The first evidence of the existence of several circulating EPCs was reported by Lin et al. Although the existence of EPCs has been demonstrated, with regard to malignant tumors the data is controversial on the pre-existing endothelium insertion rate and the extent to which these cells contribute to tumor angiogenesis. From these points of view, the results obtained so far vary between the extremely wide limits of 0 and 72 % for various human tumors. So far, no such studies have reported the contribution of EPCs in ovarian tumors. For this reason, the present study evaluated the expression of two markers, AC133 and tyrosine kinase with immunoglobulin-like and EGF-like domains 2 (Tie2), which signal the presence of EPCs in the pre-existing endothelium. In total, 62 female patients who were diagnosed with ovarian tumors were retrospectively selected over a four-year period. The patients had complete clinico-pathological and post-surgical evaluation data, and were well characterized with regard to the invasion (local and distant) and surgical protocols.

Specimens and histopathological primary processing

Tumor specimens were surgically removed and the most representative sections were carefully selected to include tumor and adjacent normal ovarian tissues. Tumor sections with necrosis and extensive hemorrhages were avoided. Small tumor tissues (10x10x3-mm biopsies) were washed in saline solution, fixed in 10% buffered formalin for 24 h and then paraffin embedded. For each paraffin-embedded specimen, 5-μm serial sections were mounted on silanized slides. One slide from each case was stained with hematoxylin and eosin using a routine method for histopathological evaluation and also for case selection for the immunohistochemical procedures. Immunohistochemistry. Heat-induced epitope retrieval was performed with a citrate-based solution (pH 6.0; Novocastra Laboratories, Ltd., Newcastle upon Tyne, UK) for 30 min. Endogenous peroxidase blocking was carried out with 3% hydrogen peroxide for 5 min, followed by incubation for 30 min with Tie2 (dilution 1:300, mouse monoclonal clone 9; Santa Cruz Biotechnology, Inc., Santa Cruz, CA, USA) and AC133 (dilution 1:300, rabbit polyclonal clone H-284; Santa Cruz Biotechnology, Inc.) as primary antibodies. The Bond Polymer Refine Detection System (Leica Biosystems, Newcastle upon Tyne, UK) was used for visualization. 3,3 Diaminobenzidine dihydrochloride was applied as a chromogen and hemotoxylin was used as a counterstain. The entire immunohistochemical procedure was performed with the Leica Bond-Max autostainer (Leica Biosystems). Upon microscopic evaluation of the hematoxylin and eosin-stained tumor specimens, four main histopathological types of ovarian tumors were identified: Serous carcinomas (62%), mucinous carcinomas (18%), clear cell carcinomas (6%) and ovarian germ cells tumors (8%) and undifferentiated carcinomas (6%). The majority of the aforementioned ovarian tumors exhibited a G2 tumor grade (58%), followed by grades G3 (39%) and G1 (3%). The immunoreaction for Tie2 was also selective for cells that defined the blood vessel lumens. Even under these conditions, a small number of vessels with Tie2-positive endothelial cells were identified in the tumor area, and the distribution model was found to be homogeneous in the small vessels (Fig. 15) and heterogeneous in the larger vessels with relatively large lumens (Fig. 15c). Unlike the reaction for AC133, Tie2 expression was positive in the endothelium of pre-existing mature blood vessels, which were larger in size (Fig. 15d). The immunoreaction was found to be restricted to the endothelium and did not stain perivascular cells. Since it was not possible to quantify the Tie2-positive cells compared with the Tie2-negative cells at the endothelial level, based on subjective observations it appears that Tie2 is less selective in identifying EPCs, and this most likely indicates the presence of pre-existing activated endothelial cells. The two cases in which AC133-positive tumor cells were identified were also Tie2-positive, but the number of positive cells was significantly higher. In evaluating AC133 and Tie2 expression, the location of the positive cells was examined and only elements with a positive cytoplasmic reaction that defined the lumens of the blood vessels were subjectively assessed. AC133 was positive in 18 out of 62 specimens (29.03%), and Tie2 was positive in 21 of the specimens (33.87%). Co-expression of the markers was noted in 17 cases (27.42%), in which it was considered that the positive reaction reflected the insertion of the endothelial progenitor cells into the pre-existing endothelium. The presence of endothelial progenitor cells did not exhibit a statistically significant correlation with vascular microdensity, vessel type or histopathological form.

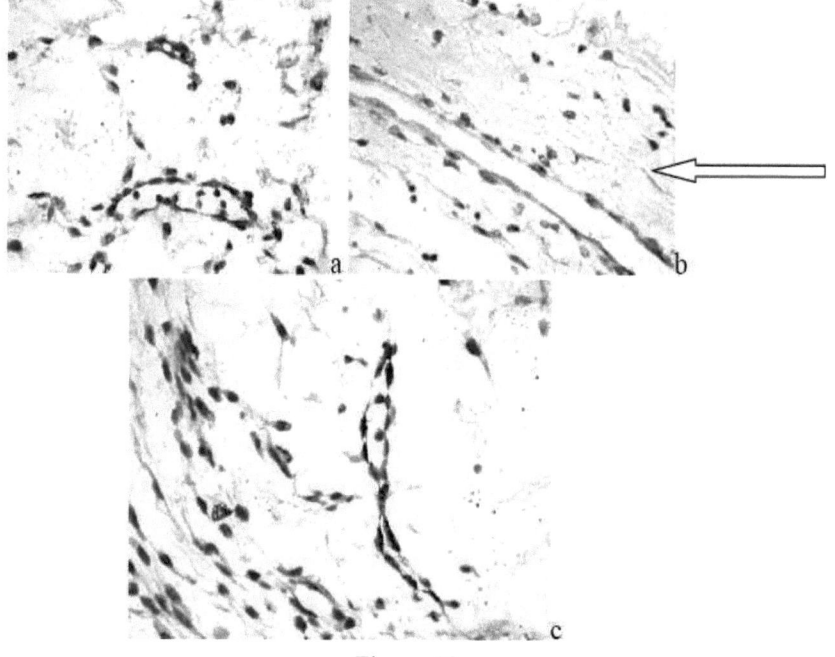

Figure 13

For the expression of AC133, the positive reaction was constantly evident in the vessels of the tumor area. These vessels were small, and relatively frequent positive endothelial cells lined the majority of the lumens (Fig. 13A). Notably, the endothelial cells were the only AC133-positive cells in the majority of the tumor stroma cases. In the peritumoral area, the blood vessels were predominantly AC133-negative, particularly when their morphology was indicative of a mature character. Occasionally, in extremely small vessels, a positive reaction was observed (Fig. 13B). The most frequently observed aspect in the intratumoral area was the heterogeneous model with alternating AC133-positive and -negative cells (Fig. 13C).

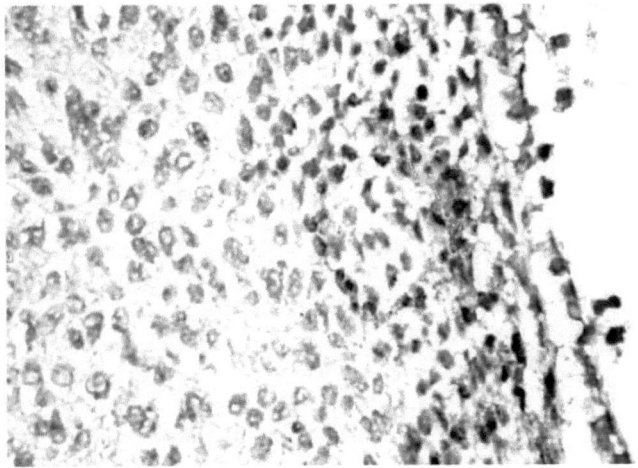

Figure 14

In only two out of the 62 cases, AC133-positive neoplastic cells were focally observed in the intratumoral area. The distribution pattern of the positive reaction was diffuse, cytoplasmic and not predominantly in the membrane (Fig. 14).

These cells formed a distinct population of tumor cells, preferentially located at the tumor proliferation front, which could represent tumor stem cells. In the present study tumor stem cells were positive for this marker, but the method of detection is not specific enough and further studies are required to demonstrate their character. The immunoreaction for Tie2 was also selective for cells that defined the blood vessel lumens. Even under these conditions, a small number of vessels with Tie2-positive endothelial cells were identified in the tumor area, and the distribution model was found to be homogeneous in the small vessels (Fig. 15) and heterogeneous in the larger vessels with relatively large lumens (Fig. 15c). Unlike the reaction for AC133,

Tie2 expression was positive in the endothelium of preexisting mature blood vessels, which were larger in size (Fig. 15d).

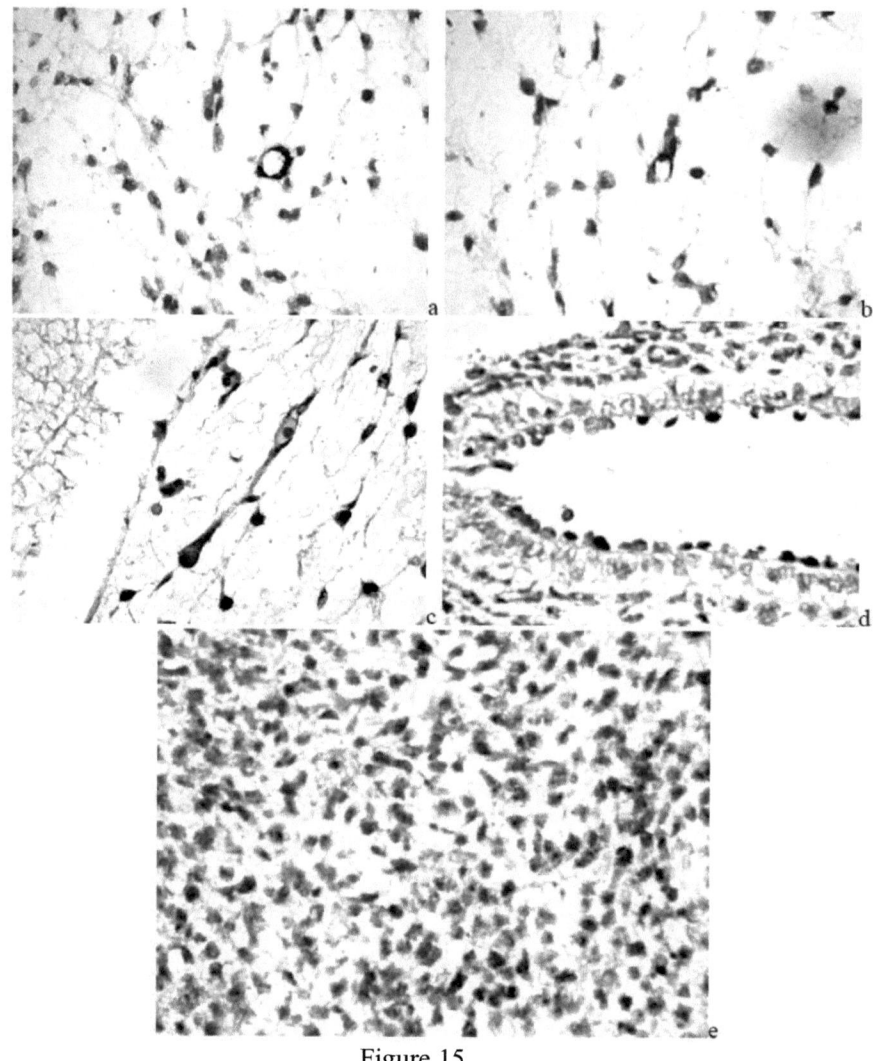

Figure 15

The immunoreaction was found to be restricted to the endothelium and did not stain perivascular cells. Since it was not possible to quantify the Tie2-positive cells compared with the Tie2-negative cells at the endothelial level, based on subjective observations it appears that Tie2 is less selective in identifying EPCs, and this most likely indicates the presence of pre-existing activated endothelial cells. The two cases in which AC133-positive tumor cells (Fig. 15e) were identified were also Tie2-positive, but the number of positive cells was significantly higher.

Tumor neovascularization represents a key point in tumor progression, and has been extensively demonstrated to result from the process of angiogenesis (Shi Q. and co., 1998). The role ascribed to the cancer cells during the process of tumor angiogenesis is the initiation of the angiogenic switch, which is a critical step in tumor progression (Grigoras and co., 2014). The tumor microenvironment plays a significant role in the activation of circulating EPCs and the mediation of neovascularization. Stressors, including hypoxia, glucose deprivation and reactive oxygen species, are activated in the tumor micro-environment and result in the upregulation of the transcription of angiogenic factors, including vascular endothelial growth factor (VEGF), stromal cell-derived factor 1 monocyte chemotactic protein-1 and erythropoietin, in EPCs (Lin and co., 2000). In the present study it was noticed that in the majority of tumor stroma cases, the endothelial cells were the only cells positive for AC133. EPCs are regarded as bone marrow-derived cells that are able to migrate into the peripheral blood in response to cytokines, such as VEGF. As opposed to in ischemic conditions, the role of circulating EPCs in tumor growth and angiogenesis is not clear. EPCs have been identified as a potential marker for the response to antiangiogenic therapies and neovascularization, and they also possess a high proliferation potential. Initially, Tie2 was found to be overexpressed in tumoral vessels, and it is also expressed in several types of cancer, including leukemia, and solid neoplasms, including gliomas and gastric and breast tumors. Tie2 expression in various tumoral compartments highlights this cellular receptor as an attractive target for cancer therapy. In summary, the results of the present study revealed that 27.4% of ovarian tumor cases express AC133 and Tie2 in blood vessel endothelial cells. The expression of these two markers did not correlate with any clinicopathological prognostic parameters, including histological type, vascular microdensity and vessel type. Co-expression of the markers most likely reflects the insertion of endothelial progenitor cells into the pre-existing endothelium. This phenomenon contributes to angiogenesis progression in cases where the budding process is reduced or absent, as shown by the inverse correlation with the rate of endothelial cell proliferation.

7. EG VEGF: A BIG DILEMMA OF THE OVARIAN CANCER

The existence of organ specific angiogenic factors has been postulated for many years and received confirmation when such a factor named endocrine gland derived vascular endothelial growth factor (EG-VEGF) was characterized and sequenced by LeCouter in 2001. The angiogenic action of EG-VEGF, appeared to be restricted to endothelial cells derived from endocrine tissues. In endothelial cells isolated from steroidogenic glands EG-VEGF was shown to promote proliferation, survival and chemotaxis (Brouillet and co., 2010). EG-VEGF also known as prokineticin 1(PROK1) is a tissue-specific angiogenic factor. Its expression is restricted mainly to the steroidogenic glands, especially to the tissues of the ovary, testis, adrenal gland, and placenta and it induces cell proliferation, migration and fenestration in capillary endothelial cells. EG-VEGF acts trough the G-protein coupled receptors prokineticin receptor 1 (PROKR 1) and prokinetikic receptor 2 (PROKR 2) which are involved in the regulation of male and female reproduction (Su and co., 2014). EG-VEGF induces the proliferation, migration and fenestration in capillary endothelial cells associated with endocrine glands, while it has little or no effect on other endothelial cells. EG-VEGF does not belong to the VEGF family, but is a member of a new protein family with multiple regulatory functions (Lin and co., 2002). Although EG-VEGF is not structurally related to the VEGF family, the biological activities of the 2 molecules are indistinguishable. These 2 major angiogenesis systems were both regulated by oxygen tension with hypoxia- inducible factor-1 alpha dependent mechanism, and were similarly hormonally regulated by estrogen, progesterone and human chorionic gonadotropin (Su and co., 2014). Angiogenesis is a major process important in both physiological and pathological conditions. EG-VEGF has been linked to several biological processes where angiogenesis is involved. EG-VEGF has been detected in the adrenal cortex, in the ovary, testis and placenta and low levels of EG-VEGF mRNA have been also demonstrated in the brain, colon, small intestine, liver, spleen and thymus. Recently, it has been shown for the first time that EG-VEGF is strongly expressed in the normal adenohypophysis (Raica and co., 2010). Evans et al 2008 demonstrated that EG-VEGF expression is elevated in human decidua during early pregnancy (Evans and co., 2008). Brouilllet et al 2010 brought further evidence that EG-VEGF is an important factor for the endothelial growth within the placental vili and participates to the development of the placenta (Brouillet and co., 2010). Su et al 2014 investigated the involvement of EG-VEGF in recurrent pregnancy loss and found that EG-VEGF plays a major in early pregnancy and may provide genetic information for the treatment of recurrent pregnancy loss (Su and co., 2014). The expression and regulation of EG-VEGF and their receptors in the human endometrium across the menstrual cycle was investigated be Battersby et al 2004. They observed a elevation of EG-VEGF expression during the secretory phase of the menstrual cycle, indicating a possible regulation by progesterone, and identified a paracrine role for EG-VEGF and their receptors in endometrial vascular function (Battersby and co., 2004). Their results were confirmed by Ngan et al 2006 who demonstrated that EG-VEGF is predominantly expressed in the glandular epithelial cells and its expression is dynamic during the menstrual cycle with a peak at the mid-luteal phase. They also stated that EG-VEGF may only play a role in vascular function of peri-implantation endometrium, but is unlikely to be associated with the development of endometrial cancer (Negan and co., 2006). As far as the normal physiology of the ovary is concerned the impact of EG-VEGF on corpus luteum was investigated by Kisliouk et al 2005. They used as model the bovine ovary and found that EG-VEGF acts as a angiogenic mitogen and survival factor for corpus luteum derived endothelial cells (Kisliouk and co., 2005). The presence of EG-VEGF has been demonstrated also in pathological conditions, such as human cancers, including ovarian carcinoma (Zhang an co., 2003), colorectal cancer (Goi and co., 2004), pancreatic adenocarcinoma (Morales and co., 2007), and benign lesions, such as polycystic ovaries (Ferrara and co., 2003). The angiogenic role of EG-VEGF is supported by the correlation found between its expression and microvascular density in all these tumors. On the other hand, the prognostic value of EG-VEGF expression by tumor cells is still a matter of debate, as no significant differences were reported between patients with high and low levels, in terms of overall survival. In addition, the clinical significance of EG-VEGF in ovarian cancer is still controversial, despite some studies found a relationship between overexpression and unfavorable prognosis.EG-VEGF expression was tested in several tumors as colon cancer, pancreatic cancer, hepatic or prostate cancer. Pasquali et al 2006 underlined that EG-VEGF could be involved in prostate carcinogenesis, probably regulating angiogenesis and suggested that the level of EG-VEGF could be useful for prostate cancer outcome evaluation and as a target for prostate cancer treatment in the future (Pasquali and co., 2006). Nagano et al 2007 investigated the expression of EG-VEGF in colorectal cancer, and found that the EG-VEGF gene functions as an important factor in angiogenesis in primary and metastatic lesions, and that EG-VEGF molecule-targeted therapy has the potential for improving survival rates (Nagano and co., 2007). Jiang et al 2008 demonstrated that EG-VEGF might act through its receptors on endothelial cells to increase angiogenesis in pancreatic diseases (Jiang and co., 2009). Li Q et al 2006 investigated the correlation between the expression of EG-VEGF along with 3 other vascular specific growth factors (VEGF, angiopoietin 2, and epinephrinB2) and carcinogenesis or portal vein tumor thrombus formation in human hepatocellular carcinoma. They found that EG-VEGF may play a role in angiogenesis and carcinogenesis of liver carcinoma by promoting portal vein tumor thrombus formation and modulating angiogenesis (Li and co., 2006). The implications of EG-VEGF signaling in human neuroblastoma progression was investigated by Ngan et al 2007. Their study indicated for the first time that aberrant EG-VEGF signaling favors neuroblastoma progression and indicated EG-VEGF as a possible target for neuroblastoma treatment (Ngan E. and co, 2007). As far as ovarian cancer is concerned the interest for antiangiogenic therapy is still very high. Due to the elevated burden of the disease new complementary treatment methods are required in order to enhance the survival rates obtained using the conventional methods: surgery and chemotherapy. Ovarian cancer is the leading cause of death from gynecological malignancies in the Western world and the majority of patients are diagnosed at an advanced stage of disease. Moreover, many cases are admitted in the stage of peritoneal spread that frequently occurs without significant symptoms. Despite the advances made in the knowledge of the genetics and molecular biology of these tumors and the effects of new chemo- therapeutic agents, its natural evolution is poorly understood. Consequently, the 5-year survival rate for patients with ovarian cancer remains low (Ramakrishnan and co., 2005). A particular aspect that was extensively investigated in patients with ovarian cancer is tumor-associated angiogenesis. There were accumulated a lot of data that support the contribution of angiogenesis to tumor cell proliferation, tumor growth and spread. In some studies, it was shown that overexpression of the vascular endothelial factor (VEGF) in ovarian carcinoma stimulates not only the formation of new blood vessels, but also induces the neoplastic transformation of epithelial cells of the ovarian surface epithelium (Bamberger and co., 2002). In clinical studies, it was shown that overexpression of VEGF is related to poor prognosis. Blockade of VEGF using humanized monoclonal antibody was thought to be a powerful therapeutic option in advanced-stage ovarian cancer, but on the other hand, results of some clinical trials based on this strategy were disappointing (Martin and co., 2007). This is explained in part by the contribution of other growth factors, like fibroblast growth factor or platelet- derived growth factor that support the proliferation of both tumor cells and endothelial cells

(Kumaran and co., 2009; Raica and co., 2010). It is more likely that angiogenesis in ovarian carcinoma is orchestrated by many growth factors and its intensity and effects on the further evolution of the tumor strongly depends on the balance between proangiogenic and antiangiogenic substances. Although many studies were conducted on ovarian cancer-related angiogenesis, the basic mechanisms of this process with this particular location remain less understood. The angiogenic role of EG-VEGF is supported by the correlation found between its expression and microvascular density in all these tumors. On the other hand, the prognostic value of EG-VEGF expression by tumor cells is still a matter of debate, as no significant differences were reported between patients with high and low levels, in terms of overall survival. In addition, the clinical significance of EG-VEGF in ovarian cancer is still controversial, despite some studies found a relationship between overexpression and unfavorable prognosis.

In the present study, we investigated the expression of EG-VEGF at protein level and we looked for a correlation with conventional parameters of prognosis in a series of patients with epithelial ovarian carcinomas. In the outer control slides, the positive reaction was restricted to the cortex of the adrenal gland and the pattern of reaction was granular cytoplasmic (not shown). In the normal ovary, the positive reaction was restricted to the covering epithelium, as a weak to moderate but homogeneous reaction. The pattern of distribution of the final product of reaction for EG-VEGF in ovarian carcinoma was mostly heterogeneous. We describe here three different models of the positive reaction in tumor cells: isolated cells that strongly express EG-VEGF, positive cells arranged in small nests, as it was particularly in the case of clear cell carcinoma , and heterogeneous. Based on the scoring system detailed above, we found an overall positive reaction for EG-VEGF in 22 cases (73.33%). From these, 14 cases were scored as +2 and eight cases as +3. An aspect with particular prognostic significance is related to the distribution of positive tumor cells at the interface between the tumor and stroma (Figure3). The number of positive tumor cells and the intensity of reaction gradually decreased in the deep tumor area. All these cases were diagnosed in the stage III and IV. We noticed a statistic significant relationship between the expression of EG-VEGF and the tumor stage (p<0.003). We also found a relationship between EG-VEGF expression and the pathological type of ovarian carcinoma.

Positive reaction was observed in 16 from 19 serous adenocarcinomas, in three from six cases with clear cell carcinoma, and in the two cases with endometrioid

47

carcinoma. All the cases with mucinous carcinoma were negative for EG-VEGF. This relation- ship was statistically significant for p<0.0001.

The intensity of EG-VEGF expression was significantly stronger in less differentiated tumors than in the others. The pattern of the final product of reaction was diffuse or heterogeneous, and the majority of tumor cells were intensely labeled. The correlation between the tumor grade and EG-VEGF expression had statistic significance (p<0.0021).

Prokineticins are a novel family of secreted peptides with diverse regulatory roles, one of which is their capacity to modulate immunity in humans and in other species (Monnier and co., 2008). EG-VEGF belongs to this family and is expressed predominantly in steroidogenic tissues (Pasquali and co., 2006). In humans, EG-VEGF expression is largely restricted to ovary, testis, adrenal cortex and placenta (LeCouter and co., 2002). This factor is certified to be involved in normal and pathologic angiogenesis (Monnier and co., 2010) and was recently reported to be responsible for the regulation of tumor cell growth and survival (Ren and co., 2009). If the angiogenic function of EG-VEGF is well established in human normal and pathologic ovary (LeCouter and co., 2004), its non-angiogenic functions is still not well characterized. In 2003, Zhang L et al. reported that EG-VEGF was undetectable by reverse transcription-PCR in 17 established epithelial ovarian cancer cell lines or in cultured human ovarian surface epithelial cells. Our results proved the EG-VEGF positive reaction in ovarian surface epithelium. This finding is in contradiction with previous ones and could explain the overexpression of EG-VEGF in all ovarian cancer, which arise from this epithelium. Also, Fraser HM et al. found a cyclic change in the expression of endocrine gland vascular endothelial growth factor in the human luteal body (Fraser and co., 2005). This could partially explain the heterogeneous expression observed in our study in ovarian surface epithelium between cases and also different EG-VEGF distribution between epithelial cells from the same ovarian surface epithelium. EG-VEGF was tested in several tumors as colon cancer (Nagano and co., 2007), pancreatic cancer (Jiang and co., 2009) or prostate cancer (Pasquali and co., 2006). Despite of the certified deep involvement of EG-VEGF in human normal ovarian physiology, expression and distribution of EG-VEGF in corresponding ovarian tumors are less mentioned in the literature (Zhang and co., 2003). We found a high overall percentage of ovarian tumors positive for EG-VEGF with three different expression patterns. Our study mentioned for the first time EG-VEGF expression patterns specifically nominated for various histopathologic types of ovarian carcinomas. Moreover, observation concerning the distribution of positive tumor cells predominantly between tumor mass and stroma strongly suggests a potential role of EG-VEGF in progression and metastasis of ovarian carcinomas. This hypothesis is supported by previous findings of Nagano et al, in colorectal carcinoma (Jiang and co., 2009). They found that its positive expression was more frequently associated with hematogenous metastasis, and was associated with poor survival rate. Other members of heparin binding growth factors family (which also include EG-VEGF) were studied in ovarian cancer as potential targets for tumor cells suppression. One of them, heparin-binding EGF-like growth factor exerts its biological activity through activation of the EGFR. Several lines of evidence have indicated that heparin binding-EGF plays a key role in the acquisition of malignant phenotypes, such as tumorigenicity, invasion, metastasis and resistance to chemotherapy (Miyamoto and co., 2006). We showed that all cases diagnosed in stage III and IV have EG-VEGF positive cells groups distributed at the periphery of the tumor, next to invasive front, and this particular aspect strongly suggests the involvement of EG-VEGF as a potential prognostic factor in ovarian carcinoma. The immunohistochemical expression of EG-VEGF in 30 patients with ovarian carcinoma showed a positive reaction in 73.33%. We found statistic significant correlation between EG-VEGF expression and stage, grade, and pathological type of the tumors. Our results support the use of EG-VEGF as a predictor of invasion and local progression as promoter of angiogenesis, and could represent an attractive therapeutic target in refractory ovarian cancer.

8. REFERENCES

1.Amis SJ, Coulter-Smith SD, Crow JC, Maclean AB, Perrett CW. Microvessel quantification in benign and malignant ovarian tumors. Int J Gynecol Cancer. 2005;15(1):58-65.

2.Asahara T, Murohara T, Sullivan A, et al: Isolation of putative progenitor endothelial cells for angiogenesis. Science 275: 964-967, 1997.

3.Bamberger ES, Perrett CW, Angiogenesis in epithelian ovarian cancer, Mol Pathol, 2002, 55(6):348–359.

4.Battersby S, Critchley H, Morgan K, Millar R, Expression and regulation of the prokineticins (endocrine gland derived vascular endothelial growth factor and BV8) and their receptors in the human endometrium across the menstrual cycle, J. Clin. Endocrinol. Metab. 2004

5.Beckers J, Herrmann F, Rieger S, Drobyshev AL, Horsch M, Hrabé de Angelis M, Seliger B. Identification and validation of novel ERBB2 (HER2, NEU) targets including genes involved in angiogenesis. Int J Cancer. 2005;114(4):590-7.

6.Benjamin, L., Hemo L, Keshet E.:Selective ablation of immature blood vessels in established human tumours follows VEGF withdrawal J. Clin. Invest. 103: 156-65, 1999

7.Boocock C., Charnock-Jones D., Sharkey A.: Expression of VEGF and its receptors in ovarian cancer: J. Natl. Cancer Inst. 87: 506-16; 1995

8.Brouillet S, Hoffman P, Benharouga M, Salomon A, Molecular characterization of EG-VEGF mediated angiogenesis: differential effects on microvascular endothelial cells, Molecular biology of the cell 2010, 21:2832-2845

9.Cao JG, Peng SP, Sun L, Li H, Wang L, Deng HW. Vascular basement membrane-derived multifunctional peptide, a novel inhibitor of angiogenesis and tumor growth. Acta Biochim Biophys Sin (Shanghai). 2006;38(7):514-21.

10.Chiyoda T, Tsuda H, Nomura H, Kataoka F, Tominaga E, Suzuki A, Susumu N, Aoki D. Effects of third-line chemotherapy for women with recurrent ovarian cancer who received platinum/taxane regimens as first-line chemotherapy. Eur J Gynaecol Oncol. 2010;31(4):364-8.

11.Chock KL, Allison JM, Shimizu Y, Elshamy WM. BRCA1-IRIS Overexpression Promotes Cisplatin Resistance in Ovarian Cancer Cells. Cancer Res. 2010 Oct 12.

12.Cimpean AM, Raica M, Suciu C. CD105/smooth muscle actin double immunostaining discriminate between immature and mature tumor blood vessels. Rom J Morphol Embryol, 2007, 48: 41-45.

13.Cîmpean AM, Raica M, Nariţa D. Diagnostic significance of the immunoexpression of CD34 and smooth muscle cell actin in benign and malignant tumors of the breast. Rom J Morphol Embryol, 2005, 46, 2: 123-130.

14.Cohen C. Image cytometric analysis in pathology. Hum Pathol. 1996;27:482-93.

15.Connolly D., Heuvelman D., Nelson R., Olander J.: Tumour vascular permeability factor stimulates endothelial cell growth and angiogenesis. J. Clin. Invest. 1989; 84: 1470-8

16.Czekierdowski A, Czekierdowska S, Danilos J, Czuba B, Sodowski K, Sodowska H, Szymanski M, Kotarski J. Microvessel density and CpG island methylation of the THBS2 gene in malignant ovarian tumors. J Physiol Pharmacol. 2008 Suppl 4:53-65.

17.Dahut WL, Lakhani NJ, Gulley JL, Arlen PM, Kohn EC, Kotz H, McNally D, Parr A, Nguyen D, Yang SX, Steinberg SM, Venitz J, Sparreboom A, Figg WD. Phase I clinical trial of oral 2-methoxyestradiol, an antiangiogenic and apoptotic agent, in patients with solid tumors. Cancer Biol Ther. 2006;5(1):22-7.

18.Darcy KM, Birrer MJ. Translational research in the Gynecologic Oncology Group: evaluation of ovarian cancer markers, profiles, and novel therapies. Gynecol Oncol. 2010;117(3):429-39.

19.Devorak H., Senger. D.: Vascular permeability factor in human tumour and inflammatory efussions , Cancer Res. 53: 2912-18,1993

20.Duff SE, Li C, Garland JM, Kumar S. CD105 is important for angiogenesis: evidence and potential applications. FASEB J, 2003, 17: 984-992.

21.Eccles SA, Massey A, Raynaud FI, Sharp SY, Box G, Valenti M, Patterson L, de Haven Brandon A, Gowan S, Boxall F, Aherne W, Rowlands M, Hayes A, Martins V, Urban F, Boxall K, Prodromou C, Pearl L, James K, Matthews TP, Cheung KM, Kalusa A, Jones K, McDonald E, Barril X, Brough PA, Cansfield JE, Dymock B, Drysdale MJ, Finch H, Howes R, Hubbard RE, Surgenor A, Webb P, Wood M, Wright L, Workman P. NVP-AUY922: a novel heat shock protein 90 inhibitor active against xenograft tumor growth, angiogenesis, and metastasis. Cancer Res. 2008 ;68(8):2850-60.

22.Evans J, Catalano R, Morgan K, Milan R, Prokineticin1 signaling and gene regulation in early human pregnancy, Endocrinology 2008

23.Fay P., Walker CJ.: Factor VIII function and structure . Thromb Haemost. 70: 63-7; 1993.

24.Ferrara N, Frantz G, LeCouter J, Dillard-Telm L, Pham T, Draksharapu A, Giordano T, Peale F, Differential expression of the angiogenic factor genes vascular endothelial growth factor (VEGF) and endocrine gland-derived VEGF in normal and polycystic human ovaries, Am J Pathol, 2003, 162(6):1881–1893.

25.Ferrara N., Gerber P.: Vascular endothelial growth factor molecular and biological aspects 237: 1-30, 1999.

26.Folkman J, Watson K, Ingber D, Hanahan D.: Induction of angiogenesis during the transition from hyperplasia to neoplasia. NEJM, 339: 58-61, 1989.

27.Fraser HM, Bell J, Wilson H, Taylor PD, Morgan K, Anderson RA, Duncan WC, Localization and quantification of cyclic changes in the expression of endocrine gland vascular endothelial growth factor in the human corpus luteum, J Clin Endocrinol Metab, 2005, 90(1):427–434.

28.Fürstenberger G, von Moos R, Lucas R, Thürlimann B, Senn HJ, Hamacher J, Boneberg EM. Circulating endothe- lial cells and angiogenic serum factors during neoadjuvant chemotherapy of primary breast cancer. Br J Cancer 2006; 94: 524-531.

29.Gadducci A, Ferrero A, Cosio S, Zola P, Viacava P, Dompé D, Fanelli G, Ravarino N, Motta M, Cristofani R, Genazzani AR. Intratumoral microvessel density in advanced epithelial ovarian cancer and its use as a prognostic variable. Anticancer Res. 2006;26(5B):3925-32.

30.Ghaemmaghami F, Hassanzadeh M, Karimi-Zarchi M, Modari-Gilani M, Behtash A, Mousavi N. Centralization of ovarian cancer surgery: do patients benefit? Eur J Gynaecol Oncol. 2010;31(4):429-33.

31.Ghosh S, Albitar L, LeBaron R, Welch WR, Samimi G, Birrer MJ, Berkowitz RS, Mok SC. Up-regulation of stromal versican expression in advanced stage serous ovarian cancer. Gynecol Oncol. 2010;119(1):114-20.

32.Giatromanolaki A, Sivridis E, Tsikouras P, Manavis I, Maroulis G, Koukourakis MI. Angiogenesis and vascular survival ability in ovarian adenocarcinomas. Virchows Arch. 2004;445(5):521-6.

33.Goi T, Fujioka M, Satoh Y, Tabata S, Koneri K, Nagano H, Hirono Y, Katayama K, Hirose K, Yamaguchi A, Angiogenesis and tumor proliferation/metastasis of human colorectal cancer cell line SW620 transfected with endocrine glands-derived-vascular endothelial growth factor, as a new angiogenic factor, Cancer Res, 2004, 64(6):1906– 1910.

34.Goodheart MJ, Ritchie JM, Rose SL, Fruehauf JP, De Young BR, Buller RE. The relationship of molecular markers of p53 function and angiogenesis to prognosis of stage I epithelial ovarian cancer. Clin Cancer Res. 2005;11(10):3733-42.

35.Gordon J., Mesiano S., Zaloudek CJ: VEGF localization in human ovary and fallopian tubes: possible role in reproductive function and ovary cyst formation; J. Clin. Endocrinol. Metab. 81; 353-9; 1996.

36.Grigoras D, Pirtea L, Ceausu A: Endothelial progenitor cells contribute to the development of ovarian carcinoma tumor blood vessels; ONCOLOGY LETTERS 7: 1511-1514, 2014.

37.Hata K, Nagami H, Iida K, Miyazaki K, Collins WP. Expression of thymidine phosphorylase in malignant ovarian tumors: correlation with microvessel density and an ultrasound-derived index of angiogenesis. Ultrasound Obstet Gynecol. 1998;12(3):201-6.

38.Hata K, Nakayama K, Fujiwaki R, Katabuchi H, Okamura H, Miyazaki K. Expression of the angopoietin-1, angopoietin-2, Tie2, and vascular endothelial growth factor gene in epithelial ovarian cancer. Gynecol Oncol. 2004 93(1):215-22.

39.Hata K, Osaki M, Dhar DK, Nakayama K, Fujiwaki R, Ito H, Nagasue N, Miyazaki K. Evaluation of the antiangiogenic effect of Taxol in a human epithelial ovarian carcinoma cell line. Cancer Chemother Pharmacol. 2004;53(1):68-74.

40.Jiang X, Abiatari I, Kong B, Erkan M, De Oliveira T, Giese NA, Michalski CW, Friess H, Kleeff J, Pancreatic islet and stellate cells are the main sources of endocrine gland- derived vascular endothelial growth factor/prokineticin-1 in pancreatic cancer, Pancreatology, 2009, 9(1–2):165–172.

41.Kaku S, Takeshima N, Umayahara K, Furuta R, Akiyama F, Takizawa K. Clinical features of 215 stage I ovarian tumors in Japanese women. Eur J Gynaecol Oncol. 2010;31(4):395-8.

42.Kamat AA, Kim TJ, Landen CN Jr, Lu C, Han LY, Lin YG, Merritt WM, Thaker PH, Gershenson DM, Bischoff FZ, Heymach JV, Jaffe RB, Coleman RL, Sood AK. Metronomic chemotherapy enhances the efficacy of antivascular therapy in ovarian cancer. Cancer Res. 2007;67(1):281-8.

43.Kawamoto A, Asahara T: Role of progenitor endothelial cells in cardiovascular disease and upcoming therapies. Catheter Cardiovasc Interv 2007, 70(4):477-484.

44.Kim K., Bing Li, Winer J., Armanini M.: Inhibition of VEGF induced angiogenesis suppresses tumour growth in vivo, Nature 362; 841-4, 1993.

45.Kim TJ, Ravoori M, Landen CN, Kamat AA, Han LY, Lu C, Lin YG, Merritt WM, Jennings N, Spannuth WA, Langley R, Gershenson DM, Coleman RL, Kundra

V, Sood AK. Antitumor and antivascular effects of AVE8062 in ovarian carcinoma. Cancer Res. 2007 1;67(19):9337-45.

46.Kisliouk T., Podlovni H., Spanel Borowsky K., Ovafia o: Prokineticins (endocrine gland-derived vascular endothelial growth factor and BV8) in the bovine ovary: wxpression and role as mitogenes and survival factors for corpus luteum derived endothelial cells, Endocrinology 2005.

47.Kumaran GC, Jayson GC, Clamp AR, Antiangiogenic drugs in ovarian cancer, Br J Cancer, 2009, 100(1):1–7.

48.Labiche A, Elie N, Herlin P, Denoux Y, Crouet H, Heutte N, Joly F, Héron JF, Gauduchon P, Henry-Amar M. Prognostic significance of tumour vascularisation on survival of patients with advanced ovarian carcinoma. Histol Histopathol. 2009;24(4):425-35.

49.Lebrin F, Goumans MJ, Jonker L, Carvalho RL, Valdimarsdottir G, Thorikay M, Mummery C,Arthur HM, ten Dijke P. Endoglin promotes endothelial cell proliferation and TGF-beta/ALK1 signal transduction. EMBO J. 2004; 23: 4018-28.

50.Lecouter J, Lin R, Ferrara N, EG-VEGF: a novel mediator of endocrine-specific angiogenesis, endothelial phenotype, and function, Ann N Y Acad Sci, 2004, 1014:50–57.

51.LeCouter J, Lin R, Ferrara N, The role of EG-VEGF in the regulation of angiogenesis in endocrine glands. In: ***, The cardiovascular system, Cold Spring Harbor Laboratory Press, 2002, LXVII:217–222.

52.Leung D.W., Cachianes G., Kuang W.J., Goeddel D.V., Ferrara N. : Vascular endolthelial growth factor is a secreted angiogenic mitogen, Science, 1989; 246: 1306-9.

53.Li B, Sharpe EE, Maupin AB, Teleron AA, Pyle AL, Carmeliet P, Young PP: VEGF and PlGF promote adult vasculogenesis by enhancing EPC recruitment and vessel formation at the site of tumor neovascularization. FASEB J 2006, 20(9):1495-1497.

54.Li Q, Xu B, Fu L, Hao X, Correlation of four vascular growth factors with carcinogenesis and portal vein tumor thrombus formation in human hepatocelular carcinoma J Exp. Clin. Cancer Res 2006

55.Lin R, LeCouter J, Kowalski J, Ferrara N, Characterization of endocrine gland-derived vascular endothelial growth factor signaling in adrenal cortex capillary endothelial cells, J Biol Chem, 2002, 277(10):8724–8729.

56.Lin Y, Weisdorf DJ, Solovey A and Hebbel RP: Origins of circu- lating endothelial cells and endothelial outgrowth from blood. J Clin Invest 105: 71-77, 2000.

57.Lin YG, Han LY, Kamat AA, Merritt WM, Landen CN, Deavers MT, Fletcher MS, Urbauer DL, Kinch MS, Sood AK. EphA2 overexpression is associated with angiogenesis in ovarian cancer. Cancer. 2007;109(2):332-40.

58.Lu C, Kamat AA, Lin YG, Merritt WM, Landen CN, Kim TJ, Spannuth W, Arumugam T, Han LY, Jennings NB, Logsdon C, Jaffe RB, Coleman RL, Sood AK. Dual targeting of endothelial cells and pericytes in antivascular therapy for ovarian carcinoma. Clin Cancer Res. 2007 15;13(14):4209-17.

59.Lu C, Shahzad MM, Moreno-Smith M, Lin YG, Jennings NB, Allen JK, Landen CN, Mangala LS, Armaiz-Pena GN, Schmandt R, Nick AM, Stone RL, Jaffe RB, Coleman RL, Sood AK. Targeting pericytes with a PDGF-B aptamer in human ovarian carcinoma models. Cancer Biol Ther. 2010;9(3):176-82.

60.Luo J, Peng ZL, Yang KX, Wang H, Yang H, Dong DD, Yao XY. Relation between the expression of hypoxia inducible factor-1alpha and angiogenesis in ovarian cancer using tissue microarray. Zhonghua Fu Chan Ke Za Zhi. 2005;40(1):38-41.

61.Mabuchi S, Altomare DA, Connolly DC, Klein-Szanto A, Litwin S, Hoelzle MK, Hensley HH, Hamilton TC, Testa JR. RAD001 (Everolimus) delays tumor onset and progression in a transgenic mouse model of ovarian cancer. Cancer Res. 2007, 15;67(6):2408-13.

62.Martin L, Schilder R, Novel approaches in advancing the treatment of epithelial ovarian cancer: the role of angiogenesis inhibition, J Clin Oncol, 2007, 25(20):2894– 2901.

63.Mc Clure N., Healy DL, Rogers PA, Sullivan J.: VEGF is detectable in the sera of tumour bearing mice and cancer patients. Biochim Biophys Acta; 1221: 211-14; 1994.

64.Merritt WM, Nick AM, Carroll AR, Lu C, Matsuo K, Dumble M, Jennings N, Zhang S, Lin YG, Spannuth WA, Kamat AA, Stone RL, Shahzad MM, Coleman RL, Kumar R, Sood AK. Bridging the gap between cytotoxic and biologic therapy with metronomic topotecan and pazopanib in ovarian cancer. Mol Cancer Ther. 2010;9(4):985-95.

65.Messiano S., Ferrara N., Jaffe R:. Role of VEGF in ovarian cancer. Am J Pathol; 153: 1249-56; 1998.

66.Minhajat R, Mori D, Yamasaki F, Sugita Y, Satoh T, Tokunaga O – Endoglin (CD105) expression in angiogenesis of colon cancer: analysis using tissue microarrays and comparison with other endothelial markers. Virchows Arch, 2006, 448: 127-134.

67.Miyamoto S, Yagi H, Yotsumoto F, Kawarabayashi T, Mekada E, Heparin-binding epidermal growth factor-like growth factor as a novel targeting molecule for cancer therapy, Cancer Sci, 2006, 97(5):341–347.

68.Mobasheri A, Airley R, Hewitt SM, Marples D. Heterogeneous expression of the aquaporin 1 (AQP1) water channel in tumors of the prostate, breast, ovary, colon and lung: a study using high density multiple human tumor tissue microarrays. Int J Oncol. 2005;26(5):1149-58.

69.Mok SC, Bonome T, Vathipadiekal V, Bell A, Johnson ME, Wong KK, Park DC, Hao K, Yip DK, Donninger H, Ozbun L, Samimi G, Brady J, Randonovich M, Pise-Masison CA, Barrett JC, Wong WH, Welch WR, Berkowitz RS, Birrer MJ. A gene signature predictive for outcome in advanced ovarian cancer identifies a survival factor: microfibril-associated glycoprotein 2. Cancer Cell. 2009 ;16(6):521-32.

70.Monnier J, Samson M, Cytokine properties of prokineticins, FEBS J, 2008, 275(16):4014– 4021.

71.Monnier J, Samson M, Prokineticins in angiogenesis and cancer, Cancer Lett, 2010, 296(2):144-149.

72.Morales A, Vilchis F, Chávez B, Chan C, Robles-Díaz G, Díaz-Sánchez V, Expression and localization of endocrine gland-derived vascular endothelial growth factor (EG-VEGF) in human pancreas and pancreatic adenocarcinoma, J Steroid Biochem Mol Biol, 2007, 107(1– 2):37–41.

73.Nagano H, Goi T, Koneri K, Hirono Y, Katayama K, Yamaguchi A, Endocrine gland-derived vascular endothelial growth factor (EG-VEGF) expression in colorectal cancer, J Surg Oncol, 2007, 96(7):605–610.

74.Ngan e, Lee K, Yeung W, Ngan HY, Ho P Endocrine glang derived vascular endothelial factor is expressed in human periimplatation endometrium, but not in endometrial carcinoma, Endocrinology 2006, 147(1):85-95.

75.Ngan E, Sit F, Lee K, Miao X, Wang W, Wong K, Garcia-Barcelo M, Implications of endocrine gland derived vascular endothelial growth factor / prokineticin -1 signaling in human neuroblastoma, Clin. Cancer Res. 2007.

76.Nilsson MB, Langley RR, Fidler IJ. Interleukin-6, secreted by human ovarian carcinoma cells, is a potent proangiogenic cytokine. Cancer Res. 2005;65(23):10794-800.

77.Nisolle M, Alvarez ML, Colombo M, Foidart JM. Endometriosis: from research to clinical practice. Bull Mem Acad R Med Belg. 2007;162(5-6):263-72.

78.O'Reilly M., Pirie-Shepherd S, Lane WS, Folkman J.: Antiangiogenic activity of the cleaved conformation of the serpin antithrombin III. Science 285: 1926-8; 1999.

79.Okamura K, Tsuji Y, Shimoji T, Miyake K. Growth of human tumor xenografts on chorioallantoic membrane of chick embryo. Hinyokika Kiyo. 1995;41(3):163-70.

80.Palmer JE, Sant Cassia LJ, Irwin CJ, Morris AG, Rollason TP. Prognostic value of measurements of angiogenesis in serous carcinoma of the ovary. Int J Gynecol Pathol. 2007;26(4):395-403.

81.Pan YL, Zheng S, Peng JP, Dong Q. Influence of microencapsulated ovary cells modified with maspin gene on the microvessel density and lung metastasis of breast carcinoma. Zhonghua Yi Xue Za Zhi. 2008;88(2):92-5.

82.Pasquali D, Rossi V, Staibano S, De Rosa G, Chieffi P, Prezioso D, Mirone V, Mascolo M, Tramontano D, Bellastella A, Sinisi AA, The endocrine-gland-derived vascular endothelial growth factor (EG-VEGF)/prokineticin 1 and 2 and receptor expression in human prostate: up-regulation of EG-VEGF/prokineticin 1 with malignancy, Endocrinology, 2006, 147(9):4245–4251.

83.Pasquali D, Rossi V, Staibano S, De Rosa G, Chieffi P, Prezioso D, Mirone V, Mascolo M, Tramontano D, Bellastella A, Sinisi AA, The endocrine-gland-derived vascular endothelial growth factor (EG-VEGF)/prokineticin 1 and 2 and receptor expression in human prostate: up-regulation of EG-VEGF/prokineticin 1 with malignancy, Endocrinology, 2006, 147(9):4245–4251.

84.Peichev M, Naiyer AJ, Pereira D, et al: Expression of VEGFR-2 and AC133 by circulating human CD34(+) cells identifies a popu- lation of functional endothelial precursors. Blood 95: 952-958, 2000.

85.Penault-Llorca F, Durando X, Bay JO. Prognostic value of epidermal growth factor receptor. Bull Cancer. 2003;90 Spec No:S192-6.

86.Peters BA, Diaz LA, Polyak K, Meszler L, Romans K, Guinan EC, Antin JH, Myerson D, Hamilton SR, Vogelstein B, Kinzler KW, Lengauer C. Contribution of bone marrow-derived endothelial cells to human tumor vasculature. Nat Med 2005; 11: 261-262.

87. Pike S., Sandra E., Yao Lei,: Vasostatin inhibits angiogenesis and suppresses tumour growth; J. Exp. Med. 188: 2349-56; 1998.

88. Pölcher M, Rudlowski C, Friedrichs N, Mielich M, Höller T, Wolfgarten M, Kübler K, Büttner R, Kuhn W, Braun M. In vivo intratumor angiogenic treatment effects during taxane-based neoadjuvant chemotherapy of ovarian cancer. BMC Cancer. 2010;10:137.

89. Raica M, Cimpean AM, Platelet-derived growth factor (PDGF)/PDGF receptors (PDGFR) axis as target for anti- tumor and antiangiogenic therapy, Pharmaceuticals, 2010, 3(3):572– 599.

90. Raica M, Coculescu M, Cimpean AM, Ribatti D, Endocrine gland derived-VEGF is down-regulated in human pituitary adenoma, Anticancer Res, 2010, 30(10):3981– 3986.

91. Ramakrishnan S, Subramanian IV, Yokoyama Y, Geller M, Angiogenesis in normal and neoplastic ovaries, Angiogenesis, 2005, 8(2):169–182.

92. Rask K, Zhu Y, Wang W, Hedin L, Sundfeldt K. Ovarian epithelial cancer: a role for PGE2-synthesis and signalling in malignant transformation and progression. Mol Cancer. 2006, 16;5:62.

93. Raspollini MR, Castiglione F, Garbini F, Villanucci A, Amunni G, Baroni G, Boddi V, Taddei GL. Correlation of epidermal growth factor receptor expression with tumor microdensity vessels and with vascular endothelial growth factor expression in ovarian carcinoma. Int J Surg Pathol. 2005;13(2):135-42.

94. Ren LN, Li QF, Xiao FJ, Yan J, Yang YF, Wang LS, Guo XZ, Wang H, Endocrine glands-derived vascular endothelial growth factor protects pancreatic cancer cells from apoptosis via upregulation of the myeloid cell leukemia-1 protein, Biochem Biophys Res Commun, 2009, 386(1):35–39.

95. Rosano L, Cianfrocca R, Spinella F, Di Castro V, Natali PG, Bagnato A. Combination therapy of zibotentan with cisplatinum and paclitaxel is an effective regimen for epithelial ovarian cancer. Can J Physiol Pharmacol. 2010;88(6):676-81.

96. Rossochacka-Rostalska B, Gisterek IJ, Suder E, Szelachowska JK, Matkowski RA, Lacko A, Kornafel JA. Prognostic significance of microvessel density in ovarian cancer. Wiad Lek. 2007;60(3-4):129-37.

97. Rubatt JM, Darcy KM, Hutson A, Bean SM, Havrilesky LJ, Grace LA, Berchuck A, Secord AA. Independent prognostic relevance of microvessel density in advanced epithelial ovarian cancer and associations between CD31, CD105, p53 status, and angiogenic marker expression: A Gynecologic Oncology Group study. Gynecol Oncol. 2009;112(3):469-74.

98.Santarelli JG, Udani V, Yung YC, Cheshier S, Wagers A, Brekken RA, Weissman I, Tse V. Incorporation of bone mar- row-derived Flk-1-expressing CD34+ cells in the endothe- lium of tumor vessels in the mouse brain. Neurosurgery 2006; 59: 374-382.

99.Schoenfeld A, Levavi H, Breslavski D, Amir R, Ovadia J. Three-dimensional modelling of tumor-induced ovarian angiogenesis. Cancer Lett. 1994;87(1):79-84.

100.Scholzen T, Gerdes J . "The Ki-67 protein: from the known and the unknown". J. Cell. Physiol. 2000; 182: 311–22.

101.Schumacher JJ, Dings RP, Cosin J, Subramanian IV, Auersperg N, Ramakrishnan S. Modulation of angiogenic phenotype alters tumorigenicity in rat ovarian epithelial cells. Cancer Res. 2007 15;67(8):3683-90.

102.Sharma R., Harris A., Dalgleish G., Steward PW.: Angiogenesis as a biomarker and target in cancer. Lancet Oncol. 2001; 726-731

103.Shi Q, Rafii S, Wu M+H, et al: Evidence for circulating bone marrow-derived endothelial cells. Blood 92: 362-367, 1998.

104.Sinh R., Interferon alpha si bata down-regulates the expression of basic fibroblast growth factor in human carcinomas. Proc. Natl. Acad. Sci. USA; 92: 4562-6; 1995.

105.Su M, Lin S, Chen C, Kuo P, Gene-gene interactions and gene polymorphism of VEGFA and EG-VEGF gene systems in recurrent pregnancy loss, J. Assist. Reprod Genet. 2014,31:699-705.

106.Sundar SS, Zhang H, Brown P, Manek S, Han C, Kaur K, Charnock MF, Jackson D, Ganesan TS. Role of lymphangiogenesis in epithelial ovarian cancer. Br J Cancer. 2006;94(11):1650-7.

107.Takahashi Y., Kitadai Y, Bucana CD: Expression of VEGF and its receptor correlates with vascularity, metastasis and proliferation of human colon cancer; Cancer Res. 55; 3964-8 ;1995.

108.Taskiran C, Erdem O, Onan A, Arisoy O, Acar A, Vural C, Erdem M, Ataoglu O, Guner H. The prognostic value of endoglin (CD105) expression in ovarian carcinoma. Int J Gynecol Cancer. 2006;16(5):1789-93.

109.Tempfer C., Obermair, A., Hefler, L., Haeusler, G.: VEGF serum concentration in ovarian cancer. Obst. Gynecol. 92 :360-3 ;1998.

110.Toi M., Hoshina S, Takayanagi T, Tominaga T.: Association of VEGF expression with tumour angiogenesis and early relapse in primary breast cancer Jpn. J. Cancer Res. 85; 1045-9,1999.

111.Tsukagoshi S, Saga Y, Suzuki N, Fujioka A, Nakagawa F, Fukushima M, Suzuki M. Thymidine phosphorylase-mediated angiogenesis regulated by thymidine phosphorylase inhibitor in human ovarian cancer cells in vivo. Int J Oncol. 2003;22(5):961-7.

112.Weidner N, Folkman J, Pozza F, Bevilacqua P, Alfred EN, Moore DH – Tumor angiogenesis: a new significant and independent prognostic indicator in early-stage breast carcinoma. J Natl Cancer Inst, 1992, 84: 1875-1887.

113.Wilkstrom P, Lissbrant IF, Stattin P, Egevad L, Bergh A – Endoglin (CD105) is expressed on immature blood vessels and is a marker for survival in prostate cancer. Prostate, 2002, 51: 268-275.

114.Wu CC, Lee CN, Chen TM, Shyu MK, Hsieh CY, Chen HY, Hsieh FJ. Incremental angiogenesis assessed by color Doppler ultrasound in the tumorigenesis of ovarian neoplasms. Cancer. 1994;73(4):1251-6.

115.Xiao-Qin Ha, Man Zhao, Xiao-Yun Li, Jun-Hua Peng, Ju-Zi Dong, Zhi-Yun Deng, Hong-Bin Zhao, Yong Zhao: Distribution of endothelial progenitor cells in tissues from patients with gastric cancer; ONCOLOGY LETTERS 7: 1695-1700, 2014

116.Xi-Tai Sun, Xian-Wen Yuan, Hai-Tao Zhu, Zheng-Ming Deng, De-Cai Yu, Xiang Zhou, Yi-Tao Ding: Endothelial precursor cells promote angiogenesis in hepatocellular carcinoma; World J Gastroenterol 2012, 21; 18(35): 4925-4933.

117.Yajuan Su, Lei Zheng, Qian Wang, Weiqi Li, Zhen Cai, Shilong Xiong, Jie Bao; Quantity and clinical relevance of circulatingendothelial progenitor cells in human ovarian cancer; Journal of Experimental & Clinical Cancer Research 2010, 29:27

118.Yancoupulos G. : Vascular endothelial growth factors and blood vessel formation, Nature 2000, 407: 242-8.

119.Zhang L, Yang N, Conejo-Garcia JR, Katsaros D, Mohamed- Hadley A, Fracchioli S, Schlienger K, Toll A, Levine B, Rubin SC, Coukos G, Expression of endocrine gland-derived vascular endothelial growth factor in ovarian carcinoma, Clin Cancer Res, 2003, 9(1):264–272.

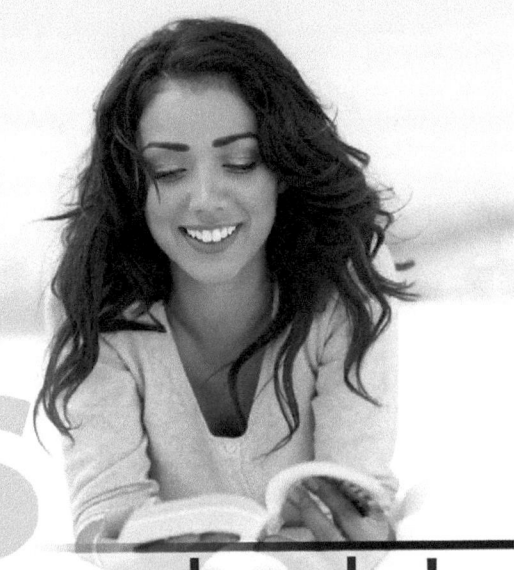
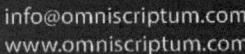
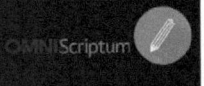

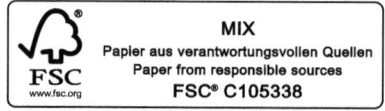